"If You Knew the Conditions"

"If You Knew the Conditions"

A Chronicle of the Indian Medical Service and American Indian Health Care, 1908–1955

DAVID H. DEJONG

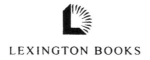

LEXINGTON BOOKS

A division of
ROWMAN & LITTLEFIELD PUBLISHERS, INC.
Lanham • Boulder • New York • Toronto • Plymouth, UK

LEXINGTON BOOKS

A division of Rowman & Littlefield Publishers, Inc.
A wholly owned subsidary of The Rowman & Littlefield Publishing Group, Inc.
4501 Forbes Boulevard, Suite 200
Lanham, MD 20706

Estover Road, Plymouth PL6 7PY, United Kingdom

British Library Cataloguing in Publication Information Available

Library of Congress Cataloging-in-Publication Data

The hardback edition of this book was previously cataloged by the Library of Congress as follows:

DeJong, David H.
  "If you knew the conditions" : a chronicle of the Indian medical service and American Indian
health care, 1908–1955 / David H. DeJong.
    p. ; cm.
  Includes bibliographical references and index.
  1. Indians of North America—Medical care—History—20th century. 2. United States.
Indian Health Service—History—20th century. 3. Indians of North America—Health
and hygiene—History—20th century. I. Title.
  [DNLM: 1. United States. Indian Health Service. 2. Delivery of Health Care—
history—United States. 3. Indians, North American—history—United States. 4. Health
Services, Indigenous—United States. 5. History, 20th Century—United States. 6.
Socioeconomic Factors—United States. WZ 80.5.I3 D326i 2008]
  RA448.5.I5D45 2008
  362.1089'97073—dc22   2008022040

ISBN 978-0-7391-2445-1 (cloth : alk. paper)
ISBN 978-0-7391-2446-8 (pbk. : alk. paper)

Printed in the United States of America

Contents

Tables

Tables

Acknowledgment

I acknowledge the friendship and support of William Katzel of Tucson, Arizona. This study began as one of his visions when we labored together at the Indian Health Service, Office of Health Program Research and Development, in Tucson. It was the wise counsel of Dr. Jennie Joe, of the University of Arizona, that put the present study in its proper perspective. Her guidance and suggestions were valuable and constructive. Finally, I acknowledge the support of my family. Cindy gave me the encouragement to persevere and my children, Rachelle, Rebecca, Joshua, Ralissa and RaeAnna, gave up precious time so that this study might be completed.

CHAPTER ONE

"If You Knew the Conditions"

On November 15, 1907, Dr. Susan La Flesche-Picotte, a member of the Omaha tribe and the first American Indian female doctor in the United States, penned a letter to Commissioner of Indian Affairs Francis Leupp. "I am an Omaha Indian and have been working as [a] medical missionary among the Omahas," La Flesche-Picotte began, "but [I] have broken down from overwork.... I know what a small figure our affairs cut with all the Department has on its hand, but I also know that if you knew the conditions and circumstances to be remedied you would do all you could to remedy them." She then described the needs of the Omaha people.

La Flesche-Piatte could have been describing the needs of any tribe in the country as, by 1907, most were approaching the nadir of their existence. "The spread of tuberculosis among my people is something terrible—it shows itself in the lungs, kidneys, abdominal track, blood, brain and glands." Recognizing the severity of the situation and the dire need for medical care, she begged Leupp "that something must be done" for the people. "The physical degeneration in 20 years among my people is terrible," La Flesche-Picotte concluded, "but I want to know if the Govt can't do for us, what it did for the Sioux in preventing the spread of the White Plague."[1]

Scores of Indians and non-Indians echoed La Flesche-Picotte's plea across Indian Country. Mary Wynkoop, a field matron from the Gila River (Arizona) Indian Reservation lamented the spread of disease among the Pima and Maricopa. "When we came to the reservation seven years ago (1896) we only knew of one case of tuberculosis among 1,500 people," she informed Commissioner William Jones. "Since that time we have buried by the scores promising young people from the schools." If Jones doubted the extent of disease, the matron encouraged him to order an examination that "would, I think, bring to light surprising results."[2]

Leupp's reply to La Flesche-Picotte is illustrative of the inability of the

Indian Service to combat disease. What medical services were provided were scattered and disjointed, with many provided by missionary agencies such as the one employing La Flesche-Picotte. "Owing to lack of funds it is quite impossible," Leupp told the physician, to do more than what is being done. American Indians represented too small a percentage of the overall population and had no voice in government affairs to protest this lack of attention. Conditions continued to decline with mortality rates rapidly rising. A library of cultural history and knowledge was dissipating, as was the loss of spiritual and political leadership in Indian Country. Demoralization, depression and discouragement were rampant in Indian Country. Many American Indians witnessed successive waves of epidemics as evidence the Great Spirit could no longer protect them. Many turned to Christianity believing the "white man's God" was more powerful.

Early U.S. Attempts to Provide Medical Care

The United States Army undertook measures to combat infectious diseases, especially smallpox, as early as 1803, although President Jefferson provided vaccinations for visiting Indian delegations to Washington, D.C. as early as 1801. This protection was largely for tribes residing near military posts along the frontier and was designed more to protect the soldiers than to ensure the health and survival of the Indians. Although some Indians were vaccinated, most were so far removed from military posts and other governmental influences that they did not receive vaccinations.

The United States also assumed responsibility for health care through the education of Indian children. The 1819 Civilization Act, enacted "for the purpose of providing against the further decline and final extinction of the Indian tribes," provided funds for education and "such other duties as may be enjoined" to protect and preserve the Indians adjoining the frontier settlements of the United States.[3] The "civilization" funds, as they were called, were administered by the Superintendent of Indian Trade and, after 1824, by the Office of Indian Affairs under the authority and at the discretion of the Secretary of War. Congress also directed such funds to be dispatched to various missionary societies, some of which provided rudimentary nursing and medical services.[4]

During the time the Office of Indian Affairs was under the auspices of the War Department (1824-1849), the dispensation of medical care was made available to small numbers of Indians living near military posts. These services were provided by army medical staff and were usually minimal, due to absence of resources for Indian health care. Where services were provided, the delivery system was inefficient, with vaccines often arriving late or not at all. Doctors remained in short supply. Indian agents frequently wrote members of Congress and officials in the War Department seeking additional funds and increased medical personnel and supplies, but usually to no avail.

When military expeditions headed into Indian Country, they were equipped with interpreters and sundry assistants but rarely with physicians to administer health services. Army Colonel Thomas McKenney, later first head of the Office of Indian Affairs, reported he personally treated (with the assistance of an interpreter) an Indian woman suffering from pleurisy because there was no physician available to accompany the troops. The only order on record concerning the health of Indians before 1832 was a War Department directive requiring "the health of the Indians to be carefully guarded" while the military removed tribes from the east to the new Indian Country in the west. When the Creek Nation removed from Georgia and Alabama in the 1830s, for example, the United States agreed to provide a surgeon to attend to the needs for each emigrating party of 1,000 people. When the Cherokee Nation was removed over the Trail of Tears, in 1838, over 4,000 men, women and children died. Smallpox was the primary cause of illness and death among the Creeks, Choctaws, Chickasaws, Seminoles and Cherokees, both during removal and upon arrival in their new lands in the Indian Territory.[5]

Not until 1832 did Congress appropriate money for Indian vaccinations and then only in response to an epidemic. An appropriation of $12,000 was made for smallpox vaccinations to save the Indians "from the destructive ravages of that disease." Secretary of War Lewis Cass was authorized to employ as many physicians or surgeons, military or civilian, as he saw fit to execute the charge. He was also charged with supplying vaccine matter to all Indian agents for "arresting the progress of smallpox among the several tribes." Using the Congressional appropriation, Commissioner of Indian Affairs Elbert Herring paid surgeons a $6 per diem or $6 per hundred vaccinations, to inoculate willing Indians in the Missouri River Valley. Herring reported to Cass that initial reports indicated when the Indians were encouraged to do so they accepted the vaccine and expressed gratitude in the efforts of the government to eliminate smallpox. Other tribes, however, especially those in Kansas and on the upper Missouri River, repeatedly resisted vaccinations due to the influence of Indian traders or their distrust of the efforts of the government. Using the meager appropriation, 10,000 Indians were vaccinated by February 1833, although the vaccination of a few thousand Indians did little to eliminate the need for health services in Indian Country.[6]

A litany of epidemics swept through the western tribes in the first decades of the nineteenth century.[7] In the summer of 1830, for instance, smallpox swept through the lower Columbia River Valley of Oregon, crippling white settlers and decimating the Indians—and this after an 1820 epidemic claimed up to 80% of the tribal people along the Colombia River. By 1833, the same plague spread into the Central Valley of California. Oregon pioneer William A. Slacum estimated some 6,000 Indians died in the Willamette Valley alone between 1830-1837. Some tribes were exterminated, "without leaving a single survivor to tell their melancholy tale." The result of the epidemic in California was nothing short of spectacular, with 20,000 Indians—or 75% of the Indian population—wiped out in just one summer. So crippled were the Indians that they could offer but little resistance to the gold-seeking 49'ers arriving just a decade and a half later.[8]

The 1830s were especially hard on the western tribes. John Dougherty, Indian agent for the Missouri River basin, wrote to Superintendent of Indian Affairs William Clark in 1831 that he had just returned from visiting four Pawnee villages, finding half of them infected with smallpox and fearing the complete annihilation of the village tribes "by the cruel and frightful" disease. Within 12 months, an estimated 4,000 Pawnees, Otoes, Omahas and Poncas had died and the disease continued spreading northward, where it reached the Winnebago. Agent Isaac McCoy exhorted Secretary of War Lewis Cass to adopt the means necessary to "arrest this destroying plague by vaccination."[9]

In 1837, smallpox swept through the upper Missouri River Valley, inflicting havoc on a trading post before sweeping through the Indian villages with horrifying results. "Language, however forcible, can convey but a faint idea of the scene of desolation, which the country now presents," Henry Rowe Schoolcraft wrote in an 1853 description of the account that killed some 10,000 Indians. An eyewitness reported, "In whatever direction you turn, nothing but sad wrecks of mortality meet the eye. Lodges standing on every hill, but not a streak of smoke rising from them." Not a sound was "heard to break the awful stillness save the numerous croaks of ravens and the mournful howl of wolves, fattening on the human carcasses that lie strewed around. It seems as if the very genius of desolation had stalked through the prairies and wreaked his vengeance on everything bearing the shape of humanity."[10]

The epidemic nearly destroyed the Mandan tribe. When it struck, the Mandans—surrounded by their hereditary enemy the Sioux—were unable to disperse upon the Plains. With their outlet to survival closed off, the Indians were forced to remain within their villages, "where the disease in a few days became so malignant that death ensued in a few hours after its attack. So slight were their hopes when they were attacked," George Catlin described, "that nearly half of them destroyed themselves with their knives, with their guns, and by dashing their brains out by leaping headforemost from a thirty foot ledge of rocks in front of their village." Catlin continued:

> The first symptoms of the disease was a rapid swelling of the body, and so very virulent had it become, that very many died in two or three hours after their attack, and in many cases without the appearance of disease upon their skin. Utter dismay seemed to possess all classes and ages and they gave themselves up in despair, as entirely lost. There was but one continual crying and howling and praying to the Great Spirit for his protection during the nights and days; and there being but few living, and those in too appalling despair, nobody thought of burying the dead, whose bodies, whole families together, were left in horrid and

loathsome piles in their own wigwams, with a few buffalo robes, etc.
thrown over them, there to decay, and be devoured by their own dogs.

When the epidemic finally ended less than 150 of the 1,600 Mandans remained
alive. A smallpox epidemic in 1838, possibly an extension of the same one that
ravaged the Plains, claimed an additional 17,000 lives in the Pacific Northwest.[11]
　　In 1849, a cholera epidemic, having originated in the east, spread up
river to St. Louis where thousands of California-bound 49'ers congregated and
from whence the disease was carried across the Great Plains and into the
Southwest. A number of tribes, principally the Sioux and Pawnee, contracted the
disease and spread it to other western tribes. When U.S. Army Captain Howard
Stansbury traveled up the Platte River, in July of 1849, he found "dead and dying"
in almost every Sioux village he encountered. The Pawnee agent estimated that
1,200 Pawnees had succumbed to the disease. The Indians had become so
frightened of the disease that they scattered in all directions, leaving the dead and
dying unattended, and spreading the disease to other villages. When a smallpox
epidemic spread through the Sioux villages in 1850, they blamed it "on white
magic designed to further their extinction."[12]

Treaty Provisions Related to Health Care

The primary means by which the United States dealt with Indian tribes before
1871 was through the treaty-making process. In exchange for hundreds of millions
of acres of land, the United States took upon itself the provision of a variety of
goods and services to the Indians. Of the 389 ratified Indian treaties, 31 (12%)
contain provisions specifically related to Indian health care: 28 providing for a
physician and 9 providing for a hospital.[13] The first treaty provision mentioning
the health of Indians was the 1832 Winnebago treaty made at Rock Island,
Illinois. Article 5 committed the United States to provide "for the service and
attendance of a physician at Prairie du Chien, and of one at Fort Winnebago, each,
two hundred dollars, per annum."[14] Other treaty provisions related to health
services were regional. In 1854-1855, for example, 14 treaties containing medical
provisions were concluded with Indian tribes in Washington, Oregon, Idaho and
western Montana. In 1867-1868, seven Peace treaties made with the tribes on the
Great Plains contained medical provisions.
　　Health facilities and physicians were increasingly important to many
tribes by the latter half of the nineteenth century. In the 1854 Chasta, Scoton and
Umpqua treaty talks, for example, Commissioner Joel Palmer reported the
government's promise to establish schools and a hospital among the Indians
"contributed very much to overcome their objections." Paternalism was also an
inducement for some tribes to sign treaties. In the 1855 treaty with the Nisqually,
Puyallup and other tribes in Washington Territory, Governor Isaac Stevens told
the Indians: "This paper is such as a man would give to his children and I will tell

you why. . . . Does not a father send his children to school? It gives you mechanics and a Doctor to teach you and cure you. Is that not fatherly?"[15]

Despite treaty provisions that provided hospitals or medical services, the United States often failed to fulfill its obligations. In the 1855 Nez Perce treaty, in which the Indians ceded a vast tract of land lying between the Cascade and Bitter Root Mountains, the United States promised "to erect a hospital, keeping the same in repair, and provided with the necessary medicines and furniture, and to employ a physician." Seven years later, however, as the government prepared to negotiate a new treaty with the Nez Perce, the United States had yet to fulfill its obligations from the 1855 treaty. "On taking charge of this Office I took pains to ascertain what had been promised to, and what had been done for the Nez Perce nation," Superintendent Calvin H. Hale reported. "I found there was not as much as you had the right to expect, not as much as the U.S. Govt supposed." Hale was "surprised to see so little improvements made, in view of the large appropriations, which I know have been made. . . . I found no hospital built . . . (because the agent) had received no money for Mills, Hospital or School." While treaties might commit funds for health care, Congressional appropriation of such funds was another matter.[16]

Treaties did not guarantee continued health care or medical staffing, since most—including several of the 1867-1868 Peace treaties—included stipulations and time limits on government supported physicians. In the 1867 Medicine Lodge Treaty with the Cheyenne and Arapaho tribes, the United States agreed to furnish the Indians with a physician but "at any time after ten years from the making of this treaty the United States shall have the privilege of withdrawing the physician." While most treaties provided stipulated limits on services, typically not to exceed twenty years, the United States adopted a policy of continuing such services under general appropriations.[17]

Post Civil War Years

By the latter decades of the nineteenth century Congress viewed the "Indian problem" as an internal domestic matter rather than a military one. Concurrently, the federal government began confining tribes on isolated reservations, compounding poor health. Cultural and dietary change forced on the sequestered Indians "naturally caused a great increase in their morbidity rate from the diseases to which they were not immune."[18] As more tribes were placed on reservations, the Indian Office sent additional administrative personnel to the agencies. With the limited number of physicians and medical provisions sent to Indian Country, the acute need for medical care only slowly became known.

In the post Civil War years the rapidity of change brought on by the rapid geographic expansion of the United States and the territorial displacement of the Indians profoundly impacted their health status. An 1867 Senate Committee assembled in the wake of the Sand Creek (Southern Cheyenne) Massacre, in eastern Colorado, provided a level of congressional understanding of the overall conditions of the Indians. Chaired by Wisconsin Senator James Doolittle, the Committee report concluded that, with the exception of the Indian Territory, the Indians were "rapidly decreasing in numbers," principally from disease, intemperance and war. Major General John Pope, a veteran of the Indian wars on the Plains, endorsed the Committee's findings, noting the Indians were "rapidly decreasing" because of poor health. Brigadier General George Wright concurred, adding tribes west of the Rocky Mountains were "rapidly diminishing by death and disease."[19]

The report slowly resonated in Washington, D.C. and in 1873 the Office of Indian Affairs undertook its first steps in organizing health care for American Indians by establishing the Division of Medicine and Education. The division was created to handle the "great need" of providing health care to the Indians. Within the new program central administrative control of the heretofore uncoordinated and sporadic Indian medical services was initiated and a rudimentary medical reporting and distribution system was implemented. Then in a reversal of policy, the Indian Office severed the education responsibilities from the Division in 1877 and abolished what was left of the health division, even though fewer than half of the Indian agencies had the services of a physician. After 1877 the Civilization Division assumed responsibility for examining monthly reports and distributing medical supplies to the agencies.[20]

The need for health services was reaching a crisis level by the 1870s. Kaw agent Cyrus Beade, describing conditions among the Kaw tribe in the Indian Territory in a letter to Commissioner of Indian Affairs Ezra Hayt, wrote "The Kaws are decreasing in number from year to year. Disease contracted with dissolute whites before their removal to Indian Territory permeates the tribe, and seems to be incurable." Two years later, Henry Mizner, agent at the Hoopa Agency in northern California, opined the Hoopa tribe was "fast being swept by disease from the face of the earth." The annual reports of the Commissioner of Indian Affairs throughout the latter nineteenth century are laced with tales of death and disease as well as requests for hospitals, physicians and medical supplies. In 1876-1877, ten separate requests were made for hospitals, with Congressional appropriations made for only one. Between 1893 and 1895, sixteen requests were made, most of which referred to the "imperative necessity" or "urgent necessity" of establishing a hospital and providing health services.[21]

Several factors precluded the delivery of adequate Indian health care throughout the latter nineteenth century, including medical degrees not being a prerequisite for employment as a physician in the Indian Office. While true of several of the states and territories as well, less than skilled physicians compounded the magnitude of Indian health problems. In 1878, C.A. Ruffee, agent at the White Earth Chippewa agency, spelled out the effects in Indian

Country. Because of unqualified doctors, many Indians lost faith in the "white man's medicine" and returned to traditional means of treating the ill. Ruffee urged Hayt to hire only medical school graduates who could prove they were competent and had "the necessary diplomas." Heretofore, the agent complained, "persons have been employed who have assumed the responsibilities of physicians and the consequences were that they met with poor success in keeping down sickness." The limited financial remuneration medical personnel received also affected the quality of Indian health care. Low salaries meant agencies had difficulty hiring or maintaining personnel. Mizner expressed such frustration when he explained he had "been unable to secure the services of a citizen physician for the salary offered ($900)."[22] As late as 1890, physicians in the Indian Service earned less than half that of their counterparts in the Army and Navy, as shown in Table 1.

Table 1

Salaries and Patient Loads for Select Federal Physician Pools, 1890

Agency	Physicians	Annual Pay*	Eligible Patients	# Treated	Per Physician
Indian	82	$1,028	180,184	68,165	831
Navy	160	$2,622	9,955	11,499	72
Army	192	$2,823	26,739	31,420	164

* Average annual salary

(Source: Commissioner of Indian Affairs, *Annual Report, 1890*, p. xxi)

Owing to the low pay and high patient loads, the Indian Service was chronically short of doctors. In 1879, 67,352 Indians were treated by a medical corps of 59 physicians—an average of 1,142 cases per physician. By 1888, when nearly the same number of Indians was treated, 81 physicians were responsible for improving the health of nearly 200,000 Indians, excluding the Cherokee, Choctaw, Chickasaw, Creek and Seminole nations (the "Five Civilized Tribes") in the Indian Territory, which maintained their own health facilities. The net result of the heavy caseloads was that physicians and, in some cases, nurses could do little more than prescribe drugs to the ill. Preventive medicine was unknown in Indian Country with some reservations having yet to receive the services of a physician.[23]

In 1890, Indian Commissioner Thomas J. Morgan supported the creation of a supervisor of Indian medical services, arguing a supervisor would facilitate Indian health services and thereby improve the quality of health care among the Indians. Agency physicians were far removed from civilization, Morgan explained, and the temptation to slight their duties was great. In the past, he had been obliged to discharge physicians for "immorality, neglect of duty, incompetency, or unprofessional conduct." With no professional associations to join, salary increases non-existent and a prohibition against physicians from maintaining a side practice (the Indian Service feared—correctly in some instances—that physicians would pay more attention to their non-Indian neighbors than to their Indian charges), retention of physicians and other competent employees was a constant challenge. With supervision by a medical expert and recognition of good service, Morgan believed, physicians would have incentives to stay, thus removing some of the barriers to practicing medicine in Indian Country.[24]

Congressional parsimony was also a challenge for the Indian Service as physicians found it futile to prescribe drugs when there was no money to acquire them. Most physicians made do without hospitals, nurses and basic medical instruments and had but few medical books. Transportation posed a significant problem, especially on large western reservations, as no financial provisions were made for wagons and teams of horses or, as one physician lamented, for "even a single horse." For some physicians any type of transportation would have made them more efficient and effective in treating Indians who were unable to come to the agency. Some agents grumbled that Congress was under the impression that the Indian Country was easily traversed with "street cars and elevated railroad lines."[25]

The United States did not begin constructing permanent hospitals for Indians until 1882. During the 1880s almost every agency physician recommended the construction of a hospital for his reservation. In 1884, seven agents requested a hospital so they could properly care for the ill. The agent at the Kiowa, Comanche and Wichita agency in western Indian Territory appealed to Commissioner of Indian Affairs Hiram Price, in 1884, stressing the treatment of the ill in their homes was less than satisfactory because the necessary medicine was rarely administered by the Indians as prescribed by the physician. Only by constructing a hospital, where the sick could be brought for proper care and treatment, could the physician be effective. An additional justification for constructing hospitals was to diminish the influence of the medicine man.

> The influence (of the medicine man) is still very great, however, and the agency physician finds it opposing him in all his practices, but especially in those cases that he is called to treat in the camps, when ... the patient is subjected to the severe treatment of the Indian doctor at the same time that the agency physician is prescribing for him. . . . I know no better way to meet this difficulty than by the building of a hospital. Not only would the physician be enabled to treat his patients more successfully, but also every Indian brought from the camp to the hospital would be thrown directly under civilizing and christianizing influences.[26]

Some agents saw hospitals as a tool to improve Indian health care. Others saw them as a means of breaking the power of medicine men.

In 1885, eight additional requests for hospitals were made, with two built—one among the Osage and one among the Menominee. By 1889, there were still just four hospitals in Indian Country, prompting Morgan to state that it was time to improve the medical services of the Indian Service and place them "on an equal footing with the medical departments of other branches of the public service." A social progressive, Morgan envisioned the development of a training program in Indian schools to instruct children in the art of nursing. A year later, he pushed for construction of a hospital in every Indian boarding school so that children could receive proper medical care. Indian nurses could also receive practical training at such facilities. In a fateful sense of irony, the commissioner lamented, the health of camp school children far surpassed that of those in the boarding schools due to poor environmental conditions of the latter. Boarding school students sent east faced climatic changes, which severely affected their health. Many children returned home from boarding school in such distress they died. The lack of government support for Indian health was, in Morgan's opinion, a "national disgrace" and without Congressional support the Indian Service was "powerless to remedy a great evil."[27]

A Slow Transition

By the turn of the twentieth century, there were only five Indian hospitals, although there remained Indians who, for cultural or religious reasons, refused to avail themselves of services. Many Indians had little interest in receiving care from doctors they perceived as impersonal and who treated the body without considering the mind and soul. Z.T. Daniel, physician at the Pine Ridge agency, in 1894, noted the cultural challenges facing Indians in seeking hospital treatment.

> In old times they destroyed all buildings and tepees in which a death occurred, which idea they still adhere to but seldom execute now. . . . They have an aversion to being sick in a house where a corpse has lain. Then, too, they are intensely social, and in a hospital their visitors are not so numerous, nor are the patients and visitors allowed to gormandize, as is their custom in the camp. The patient is put on a sick diet, which, to him, is synonymous with starvation. They are under restraint in everything in a hospital. There can be no drumming, incantations, songs, etc, . . . no vociferous proclamations of the sickness . . . no wailing by old crooning women. . . . It is too quiet, too still, too mysterious; it is another world to them, and they dislike everything about a hospital; their attention is continuously fixed on the deaths and failures. An Indian policeman one day was sick and applied for treatment. I suggested that he go into the hospital: He replied, 'No, that is the dead home.'[28]

Tribal shaman and traditional healers continued to exercise a level of influence over the people, encouraging them to remain faithful to their traditional ways. But even if all American Indians had accepted the "white man's" medicine, there were not enough physicians, too few hospitals and insufficient medical supplies to improve their collective health status. Nonetheless, the federal government sought to persuade resistant Indians to accept the new medicine. On ration days and other special occasions, agency physicians put on medical exhibitions in front of the Indians, showing how quickly they could extract bad teeth, lance boils or perform minor surgical operations.[29]

Because many elderly Indians refused treatment, children presented the Indian Service with its greatest hope for cultural conversion. T.D. Howard, physician at the Green Bay Menominee agency, explained it was "with the children that we get our best results, since they are easily managed and respond more quickly." Not surprisingly, the Indian Service focused most of its attention on educating Indian children and through them hospitals in Indian Country gained wider acceptance as evidenced by the number of Indian school hospitals built after 1900.[30]

With anemic appropriations preventing the construction of Indian hospitals, disease continued to ravage Indian Country. In 1898-1899, smallpox struck the Pueblo Indians, claiming 249 lives among the Zuni alone. The spread of the disease illustrates the challenges facing organized health services in the latter nineteenth century. When smallpox was first detected in 1897, the Pueblo agent received and distributed 3,000 vaccine points, later requesting an additional 5,000. Most of the points were worthless, stirring the passion of the agent, who wrote to Commissioner William Jones "this epidemic proves that the responsibility rests with the utter worthlessness of the vaccine points furnished to this agency." Of the 1,000 vaccinations made in Zuni Pueblo only a handful proved effective.[31]

To prevent the spread of the disease, each Pueblo Governor was ordered to disallow his people to visit other pueblos. Any Indian found traveling without proper authorization was to be arrested. Despite efforts to contain it, smallpox managed to work its way west to the Hopi villages where, in December of 1898, it surfaced in the First Mesa village of Walpi. Although vaccinations and quarantines were employed to prevent the spread of disease, it broke out in rapid succession and spread to all Hopi villages on First and Second mesas. With traditional Hopis refusing help—and with transportation up to Second Mesa almost impossible—the disease ran unimpeded. By the time it was brought under control, 187 Hopis had died. Of 632 cases on First and Second Mesas, 412 patients submitted to vaccinations. Of these 24 (6%) died; of the 220 traditionalists who refused treatment, 163 (74%) died. Similar outbreaks occurred in the Indian Territory.[32]

The deficiencies in Indian health could no longer be overlooked and charges were leveled against the Indian Service for neglecting Indian health care. The situation in Indian Country could hardly be considered a crisis, however, as the Indian Service had no reasonable idea of the extent of disease since it lacked any meaningful epidemiological statistics upon which to chart a plan of action. This only added to the rising chorus of critics who charged the Indian Service with benign neglect. Among the more vocal critics was Indian inspector William J. McConnell who spent most of his four-year term (1897-1901) investigating neglected Indian health needs. McConnell especially lamented the policy of filling Indian boarding schools at all costs, even if it meant admitting diseased children. The inspector wrote Interior Secretary Ethan Allen Hitchcock in 1899, that the United States had declared war on Spain because of its harshness towards the Cubans. "Yet," McConnell boldly asserted, "I venture to say that upon every one of our Indian Reservations in the Northwest there are conditions as bad or worse than any which were exposed in Cuba."[33] Spurred on by McConnell and others like him, the Indian Office slowly began expanding health facilities and paying better attention to the unhealthful overcrowding of Indian boarding schools. While there were five Indian hospitals in 1900, there were 50 by 1911. The number of physicians doubled from 85 in 1900 to 196 by 1918, as shown in Table 2.

Table 2

Hospitals and Medical Personal, Select Years, 1888-1918

Year	Hospitals	Physicians	Nurses	Matrons
1888	4	81	0	0
1895	4	74	8	3
1900	5	83	27	21
1918	87	196	99	87

(Source: *The Indian Service Health Activities*, 1922)

The number of nurses and field matrons also increased after 1900. Field matrons, first employed by the Indian Service in 1891, were in a role similar to that of a visiting county nurse and were of some value in teaching preventive health measures, such as basic sanitation and hygiene. They soon earned for themselves the name Good Samaritans of the Indian Service. Nurses first appeared in the Indian Service in the 1890s and were more directly involved in treating the ill. Nurses prior to 1900 were employed in the Indian boarding schools.[34]

The Indian Service to its credit took a creative approach in its attempt to deal with the health care morass in which the American Indians found themselves. After Congress enacted into law the General Allotment Act of 1887, an act designed to emancipate the Indians from the "bonds" of tribalism by allotting land to individual Indian landowners, the Indian Service pushed the construction of so-called "civilized" houses in place of traditional Indian dwellings. In 1905, Indian Commissioner Francis Leupp ordered Indian agents and employees of the Service to encourage home-building, arguing "Indians who set up tepees have no feeling of the American word 'home'." Assistant Commissioner Edgar Meritt urged Congress to use individual Indian trust funds to build every Indian a new home as a means of combating disease. If trust funds were not available, Meritt recommended the sale of surplus land to provide the means of constructing new homes. While the Indian Service did not expect the Indians to immediately accept "civilized" housing, it did expect them to do so sooner than later—even when doing so led to a higher incidence of disease and epidemics of a greater magnitude.[35]

The majority of Indians had never lived in permanent housing, making the transition from traditional to non-traditional houses difficult and, at times, deadly. Many Indians had a limited understanding of contagion and hygiene in a permanent home, having lived for centuries in dwellings that were frequently moved or burned and not as susceptible to disease. Dr. George M. Kober, for example, noted that during his twenty-year tenure in the United States Army (1874 to 1894) he had not encountered a single case of pulmonary tuberculosis among the Paiutes near Fort McDermitt, Nevada, until after 1884, "and then only among Indians who had exchanged their tepees for badly constructed and insanitary dwellings." George E. Bushnell, given medical charge of 2,800 Sioux prisoners of war in 1881, observed those Sioux residing near the agency were more prone to disease and illness than those not confined to permanent dwellings.

> Here was the mingling of two streams, the one kept free of the diseases of the whites, by enforced separation through continuous warfare; the other contaminated by the diseases and vices of civilization. The writer has frequently seen the scrofulous youths from the agency, their fleshless limbs fully clad, looking on wistfully at the dances of the warriors in the summer twilight, where braves, stripped to the breech-clout, danced on the grass to the music of the tom-tom, reproducing, in pantomime, their exploits in border warfare, or in some horse stealing, and revealing in many instances a magnificent physique and a boundless vitality, which contrasted cruelly with the listless aspect of some of their spectators. The two streams became one, when the Indians abandoned their tepees and took up their residence in houses under guidance of the agency officials. [36]

The introduction of "civilized" housing among the Red Lake Chippewa proved equally destructive when a tuberculosis epidemic broke out shortly after the turn of the twentieth century. While traditional Chippewa homes were temporary, clean and moved periodically for sanitary reasons, their new homes were small, log-framed, permanent dwellings with narrow windows, poor ventilation and insufficient light. Poor ventilation and lighting resulted in stagnate air, which quickly became a breeding ground for disease. In 1906, Leupp was informed of the need to advise the tribe about the necessity of receiving adequate amounts of sunlight and proper ventilation. The advice arrived too late as an epidemic swept across the reservation with the outbreak corresponding "with the introduction and proliferation of 'civilized' housing." Nearly one-fourth of the tribal members suffered from the epidemic, "which was spread by close personal contact in overcrowded, poorly constructed and ventilated, non-traditional dwellings." In 1910, Congress appropriated funds for the construction of a tuberculosis sanitarium at Red Lake. A similar outbreak of disease occurred among the Rosebud Sioux.[37]

A Crisis Unknown

Shortly after the turn of the twentieth century, Dr. Laurence W. White, superintendent of the Lac du Flambeau (Wisconsin) Indian School opined to participants at the annual Lake Mohonk Conference that the health maladies affecting American Indians were to a large measure the direct responsibility of the United States Government, which forced changes on the Indians without preparing them ahead of time. The Indian, White reported, "was taken from a domain as large as the continent itself and compelled to occupy very restricted areas before he was taught the proper rules of sanitation." Dietary changes "to which he was not accustomed" were forced on him before he had "a knowledge of how properly to prepare it." Being "forced into a new world and compelled to live a new life without a rule or law yet learned by which he might adjust himself to his new surroundings," the American Indians struggled to survive. Other humanitarians recognized the real "white plague" in Indian Country was "the vices of the white men" perpetrated on Indians by the less than scrupulous.[38]

These same events occurred throughout Indian Country in the final decades of the nineteenth century, resulting in widespread illness. The rapid push to "civilize" the Indians not only took its toll in a decreasing land base and displaced political and social structures but more importantly in the further decline of the Indians' health. Poor housing and susceptibility to successive waves of disease created a health crisis in Indian Country that the Indian Service poorly understood. The population of American Indians continued to decline, dropping from 600,000 to about 250,000 over the course of the nineteenth century. When the population dropped still further after 1900, American Indians came to be viewed as a "vanishing race."

It was in this context that La Flesche-Picotte wrote Leupp for assistance, in 1907. The physician encouraged Leupp to consider new approaches to the health challenges facing Indian Country. Within months, Leupp contacted national tuberculosis expert Joseph Murphy to head up and organize an Indian medical service. While not the first attempt to organize medical services for American Indians, the 1908 effort marked the beginning of permanent medical services in Indian Country. These services would continued within the Indian Service (modern Bureau of Indian Affairs) until 1955, when Congress transferred the Indian health program into the more capable and better organized Public Health Service. This chronicle specifically examines the history of Indian health care and services from 1908 until the creation of the Indian medical service in 1955 when the medical division was transferred into the United States Public Health Service. Table 3 below provides a chart of the Directors of the Indian medical service between 1908-1955.

Table 3

Directors of the Indian Medical Service, 1908-1955

Name	Years of Service
Joseph A. Murphy	1908 - 1918
Robert E.L. Newburne	1918 - 1926
Marshall C. Guthrie	1926 - 1933
James G. Townsend	1933 - 1941
J.R. McGibony	1941 - 1945
Ralph B. Snavely	1945 - 1948
Fred T. Foard	1948 - 1952
Burnet M. Davis*	1952 - 1953
James R. Shaw**	1953 - 1955

*Acting Medical Director
**Shaw remained as director after the transfer, retiring in 1962

Notes

1. Handwritten letter from Dr. Susan La Flesche-Picotte to Commissioner of Indian Affairs Francis Leupp, dated St. Vincent's Hospital, Sioux City, Iowa, November 15, 1907, Office of Indian Affairs, Letters Received, File 162, no. M90863, National Archives and Records Service.

2. Commissioner of Indian Affairs, *Annual Report*, "Report of Field Matron, Pima Agency, dated August 15, 1903," (Washington, DC: GPO, 1903), 135.

3. 3 Stat. 516.

4. Ruth M. Raup, *The Indian Health Program 1800-1955* (Washington, DC: GPO, United States Department of Health, Education and Welfare, Public Health Service, 1959), 1

5. *Tuberculosis among the North American Indians: Report of a Committee of the*

National Tuberculosis Association (Washington, DC: GPO, 1923), 92-93; Commissioner of Indian Affairs, *Annual Report* (Washington, DC: GPO, 1892), 299; See also "The Indian Service Health Activities," (Office of Indian Affairs, Bulletin 11), 1922. The latter argues that physicians were employed "more for the benefit of Government agents than for Indians;" Grant Foreman, *Indian Removal* (Norman: University of Oklahoma Press, 1932), 110, 184-185 and 222-223. Foreman notes that out of 1,600 Creeks who left for the Indian Territory on March 20, 1837, 177 died by August 1.

      6. "An Act to provide the means of extending the benefits of vaccination, as a preventive of small-pox, to the Indian tribes, and thereby, as far as possible, to save them from the destructive ravages of that disease," 4 Stat. 514; Elbert Herring to Lewis Cass, January 31, 1833, in "Letter from the Secretary of War, transmitting a report of the Commissioner of Indian Affairs in relation to the execution of the act extending the benefit of Vaccination to the Indian Tribes, &c," February 2, 1833, *House Document no. 82*, 22nd Congress, 2nd session (Washington, DC: GPO). The vaccine points were sent by mail to the agencies but much of it was bad, requiring the agents to purchase new vaccine points. Herring argued there were many unvaccinated tribes that were interested in vaccinations. "Small Pox among the Indians, Letter from the Secretary of War on the Subject of the Small Pox among the Indians," *House Document no. 51*, 25th Congress, 3rd session, (Washington, DC: GPO). Commissioner T. Hartley Crawford wrote to Secretary J.R. Poinsett on December 14, 1838, that small pox had yet to be arrested on the Upper Missouri River largely due to apathy on the part of the Indians. There were 10,145 vaccinations distributed as follows: Sioux 3,000; Potawatomie and Miami 86; Indians of Illinois 513; Sioux 665; Osage 2,177; Shawnee and Kickapoo 1,645; Chippewa and Ottawa 2,070. Cass sent a circular letter to all Indian agents in Illinois and Michigan requiring them to explain the vaccination process to the Indians, a feat that would require "some time and perseverance." "Memorial of Sylvanus Fansher praying for the Establishment of a permanent vaccine institute for the benefit of the army, navy and Indian Department," April 18, 1838, in *Senate Document no. 385*, 25th Congress, 3rd session, (Washington, DC: GPO).

      7. Epidemics, of course, struck hard in the east as well. See Russell Thornton, *American Indian Holocaust and Survival: A Population History Since 1492* (Norman: University of Oklahoma Press, 1987); Henry F. Dobyns and William R. Swagerty, *Their Numbers Became Thinned* (Knoxville: University of Tennessee Press, 1983); Henry F. Dobyns, "Native Historic Epidemiology in the Greater Southwest," *American Anthropologist* 91, no. 1 (March 1989); Sherburne F. Cook, "Disease and Extinction of New England Indians," *Human Biology* 45, no. 3 (September 1973); Dean R. Snow and William A. Starna, "Sixteenth Century Depopulation: A View from the Mohawk Valley," *American Anthropologist* 91, no. 1 (March 1989); Alfred Crosby, "Virgin Soil Epidemics as a Factor in the Aboriginal Depopulation in America," *William and Mary Quarterly* 3, no. 33 (April 1976).

      8. Sherburne W. Cook, "The Epidemic of 1830-1833 in California and Oregon," in *University of California Publications in American Archaeology and Ethnology* (University of California: Berkeley, 1950), 315, 322.

      9. Dougherty to Clark, dated October 29, 1831, Cantonment Leavenworth, in "Smallpox among the Indians, Letter from the Secretary of War upon the Subject of the

Small Pox among the Indian tribes," *House Document no. 190*, 22nd Congress, 1st session, (Washington, DC: GPO) March 30, 1832, 1-2. Dougherty told Clark the Indians "were dying so fast, and taken down at once in such large numbers, that they had ceased to bury their dead, whose bodies were to be seen, in every direction, laying about the river, lodged in the sand bars, in the hog weed around their villages, and in their corn caches; others again were dragged off by the hungry dogs onto the prairie, where they were torn to pieces by the more hungry wolves and buzzards. Their misery was so great and so cruel, that they seemed to be unconscious of it, and to look upon the dead and dying as they would on so many dead horses." Isaac McCoy to Lewis Cass, dated Strother's Hotel, Washington, DC: March 23, 1832, and March 27, 1832, 2-3.

10. Henry Rowe Schoolcraft, *Information Respecting the History, Conditions and Prospects of the Indian Tribes of the United States*, (Philadelphia, 1853), 1:258.

11. Cited in Crosby, "Virgin Soil Epidemics," 298-299.

12. Wilcomb E. Washburn, *The Indian in America* (New York: Harper and Row, 1975), 106. European-induced epidemics were undoubtedly more numerous than has been demonstrated. As colonists and explorers went west, the interior and western tribes who had yet to experience European diseases fell victim to epidemics. The Blackfeet, for example, succumbed to numerous epidemics—smallpox in 1781, 1837-1838, 1849-1850, and 1869-1870; scarlet fever in 1837; and measles in 1864-1865. There were scores of epidemics that spread throughout the interior of the continent far ahead of the advancing frontier that were never documented and therefore lost from the historical record. There has never been a systematic collection of tribal oral tradition describing the effects of such epidemics, although they are undoubtedly preserved in the oral tradition of many tribes. See Robert Boyd, *The Coming of the Spirit of Pestilence* (Vancouver, British Columbia: University of British Columbia Press, 1999), 22-24.

13. Most other treaties provided assurances of United States protection, which has generally been interpreted to mean that the United States would provide the means to preserve the health of the Indians. This legal framework, along with federal court rulings and legislation, forms the basis of the federal-Indian trust relationship.

14. The Winnebago treaty is found at 7 Stat. 370, at 372.

15. National Archives, Record Group 75, Microcopy T-494, *Ratified Treaties 1854-1855*, Roll 5, frames 155, 294.

16. 12 Stat. 957. National Archives, Record Group 75, Microcopy T-494, *Ratified Treaties, 1856-1863*, roll 6, frame 677, 187.

17. 15 Stat. 593.

18. J.G. Townsend, "Indian Health-Past, Present and Future," in Oliver LaFarge, editor, *The Changing Indian*, (Norman: University of Oklahoma Press, 1942), 30.

19. "Condition of the Indian Tribes: Report of the Joint Special Committee appointed under Joint Resolution of March 3, 1865," *Senate Report no. 156*, 39th Congress, 2nd session, (Washington, DC: GPO, 1867), 3-4.

20. *The Indian Service Health Activities*, 1.

21. Report of the Commissioner of Indian Affairs, *Annual Report*, 1877 (Washington, DC: GPO), 94. *Annual Report*, 1879, 9.

22. *Annual Report*, 1878, 79; 1879, 9.

23. *Annual Report*, 1888, xxxv.

24. *Annual Report*, 1890, xx.

25. *Tuberculosis among the North American Indians*, 95.

26. *Annual Report*, 1884, 81.

27. *Annual Report*, 1889, 14; 1890, xxii; 1894, 290; 1892, 63. See David H. De-Jong, *Promises of the Past: A History of Indian Education in the United States* (Boulder, Colorado: North American Press, 1993).

28. *Annual Report*, 1894, 290.

29. *Tuberculosis among the North American Indians*, 93.

30. *Annual Report*, 1893, 344.

31. *Annual Report*, 1899, 249.

32. Robert A. Trennert, "White Mans Medicine vs. Hopi Tradition: The Smallpox Epidemic of 1899," *Journal of Arizona History* 33, no. 4 (Winter 1992): 349-366. For the outbreak in the Indian Territory see, "The Relief of Certain Indians," Letter from the Secretary of the Treasury, dated July 30, 1909, *Senate Document no. 148*,61st Congress, 1st Session (Washington, DC: GPO: 1909).

33. McConnell to Secretary of Interior, February 20, 1899, Letters Received Office of the Secretary of the Interior, Official Letters of W.J. McConnell, National Archives, Record Group 48.

34. *The Indian Service Health Activities*, 5, provides a brief overview of the duties of matrons.

35. *Annual Report*, 1905, 404; Edgar Meritt, "Sanitary Homes for Indians," *The Red Man*, (Carlisle Indian School Publication), 4:10, June 1912, 445; See also Meritt, "Health Conditions among Indians," *The Red Man*, (Carlisle Indian School Publication). 6:9, May 1914, 347.

36. *Tuberculosis among the North American Indians*, 8, 10.

37. Richard Sense, "The Transformation of Chippewa Life on the Red Lake Reservation, Minnesota: 1863-1921," (Unpublished research paper, University of Arizona, American Indian Studies Department Library, 1989), 32.

38. *Tuberculosis among the North American Indians*, 42. George P. Donehoo, "The White Plague of the Red Man," *The Red Man*, 5, no. 1, 416. Donehoo also traces the history of Indian-white health exchanges.

CHAPTER TWO

Organizing the Indian Medical Service

In 1914, Warren K. Moorehead summed up the crisis in Indian Country: "That the Indians of the present are in a deplorable condition as to health no person familiar with Indian affairs will deny. It is incomprehensible to me that appropriations for combating disease are so meager, and the appropriations for allotting and education so lavish." An anonymous critic went to the heart of the crisis. "Of what use is education to an Indian with consumption? An Indian child learns to read and write, contracts trachoma, is sent home and goes blind. How does that education benefit the blind Indian?" Haven Emerson, President of the American Indian Defense Association and Director of the Institute of Public Health at Columbia University, called the Indian Service "the most disgraceful apology of scientific or humane medical care" in the country.[1]

At the turn of the twentieth century, new studies indicated that the main causes of disease in Indian Country were environmental, with Indian schools one of the prime conveyors of ill-health. While Indian Commissioner Thomas Morgan (1889-1893) labored to establish an efficient Indian school system, commissioners Daniel Browning (1893-1897) and William Jones (1897-1905) encouraged superintendents to fill schools by making a "thorough canvass of the reservations" so that eligible Indian children were enrolled. In so doing, schools designed to prepare youth for modern life became the cause of their morbidity.[2]

A Chorus of Criticism

The Indian Service faced criticism from all directions after the turn of the twentieth century. L. Webster Fox, an outspoken physician from Philadelphia, expressed a common view when he noted, "the work of the Indian Service does not make a good showing." Having evaluated trachoma among the Blackfeet tribe in Montana, Fox determined 351 out of 1,168 Indians had the disease. If such conditions existed in New York City, Fox opined, "health authorities would begin to show considerable industry in eradicating it rather than give an historical review of their manifold activities dating back to 1888," as the Indian Service had recently done. Another critic simply stated the "medical situation is as deplorable as it is disgraceful." Charles Lummis, a popularly read Indian reformer, argued it was apparent that taking children from western tribes to attend school in the east could "have but one effect—[high morbidity and mortality rates]. That is no theory."[3]

Medical anthropologist Washington Matthews shared Indian health conditions with the scientific community at every opportunity. Indian Inspector William McConnell was instrumental in the Indian Service facing up to the challenges of tuberculosis. While examining a San Carlos Apache school in Arizona Territory, McConnell decried the government's policy of filling such schools at all costs. Students were "superficially examined and others not at all," McConnell informed Interior Secretary Ethan Allen Hitchcock. "Tuberculosis frequently develops, and apparently for no other reason than to maintain a full attendance, they are kept until the last stage [of the disease] is reached." To prevent deaths from occurring at school, students were "carted home, to their tepe (sic), where in some instances even a few days suffices to bring the end. In this manner the disease is disseminated among the pupils in the schools, and the few days they occupy the home tepe may be, and no doubt is, frequently the cause of the other members of the family becoming affected."[4]

Visiting the Blackfeet, McConnell found that two, and often three, school children shared a single bed—with one pillow. "No child sleeps alone," McConnell wrote Hitchcock. "Among the children thus packed away are sandwiched in cases of both pulmonary and lymphatic tuberculosis." Out of fifteen Shoshone boys sent to Carlisle Indian School, eleven died there or soon after arriving home. "The word murder is a fearful word," the inspector announced, "but yet the transfer of pupils and subjecting them to such tearful mortality is little less." Inspector Frank Armstrong, in a letter to Hitchcock, decried the lack of physicians in Indian Country. While at the Quinaielt Reservation in Washington State, Armstrong informed the secretary that the Indians "have frequent need" for physicians. When someone was ill, it took three or four days for a contract physician to arrive, often too late.[5]

Outside the schools, conditions were little better. Agency physicians were often at odds with the Indian agent or superintendent over medical matters. Dr. L. Breen of Fort Lewis, Colorado, chastised the Indian Service for granting Indian agents authority to control the dispensation of medical supplies. This ought not to be, Breen told Jones. At no time should the agent "be allowed to interpose his opinion against the opinion of the [physician or] medical supervisor." Physicians required such authority and to insure they had it, a medical division was fundamental. Dr. Joseph G. Bullock, of the Oneida (Wisconsin) Indian School, unsuccessfully sought to organize an Indian medical service in 1898, using the conditions in the Indian schools as his primary justification.[6]

With charges of overcrowded schools and admitting contagious students, Jones was compelled to respond. In a circular sent to all agencies and schools, Jones declared war upon "dust, filth, foul odors, and all disease breeding spots." Schools were to be filled to capacity but with healthy children. "There must, most positively, be *no overcrowding* in the dormitories to the detriment of the children sleeping in them. If you have an insufficient number of healthy children to fill up your school, do not place any more therein." Indian children were to be educated, not incapacitated. The care of the students was to be "strictly enforced."[7]

The Indian Health Survey of 1903

The physical environment in the Indian schools changed the way the Indian Service viewed health matters. In its 1884 *Regulations for the Indian Department*, the Indian Service made no mention of health care or conditions. Within a decade the department took notice and instructed physicians to improve sanitary and hygienic conditions and to instruct Indian students to do the same. While regulations changed on paper, most medical activities by necessity focused on the convalescing or the treatment of disease, rather than its prevention. Facing charges of outright neglect, Jones initiated the first comprehensive health survey of Indian schools and reservations.[8]

Jones ordered all Indian Service physicians to make detailed statistical reports on the health conditions of adult Indians, students returned from off-reservation schools and local non-Indian communities. Under Indian Service Circular 102, physicians tabulated death rates, examined the conditions of buildings in relation to disease, and identified other pertinent information that impacted the health and well-being of the Indians. What Jones discovered was that conditions were far worse than he cared to admit. Tuberculosis was more widespread among Indians than among non-Indians, even though many Indians lived in regions that were considered unfavorable for the development of the disease (i.e., the Southwest).

The causes of disease were largely cultural and environmental. Poor sanitation, failure to disinfect tubercular sputum, improper diets, lack of proper medical attention, alcoholism, taking children predisposed to tuberculosis from camp life and confining them in crowded schoolrooms and dormitories, and a general biological weakening of the American Indian were factors. The sordid conditions in which many Indians lived and their cultural views of health care— euphemistically labeled "superstitions"— were important causal factors.

Trachoma and other eye diseases were also rampant. Like tuberculosis, the causes of trachoma were mostly environmental. Mitigating personal uncleanliness and neglect of simple eye inflammations was essential to improving the status of Indian health, both on an individual and collective basis. Jones concluded the health and welfare "of the Indian is and always must be the fundamental consideration in any scheme to educate or civilize him." The government had no right to deprive the Indians of ordinary health, as it was impossible to "develop his mental and moral capabilities without healthy material to work on."[9]

With the study in hand, the commissioner sent a circular letter to all Indian schools and agencies outlining additional regulations to improve Indian health. Physicians were required to thoroughly examine all prospective students before admitting them to school. Any child with symptoms of tuberculosis was prohibited from enrolling. Periodic checks were to be made to determine if a child contracted any symptoms of the disease. Since floating dust particles easily diffused tuberculosis, school superintendents were ordered to clean all dormitories and insure they received adequate sunlight. Physicians were instructed to provide weekly discourses on hygiene to students. To prevent eye disease, students were to receive prompt care and all reasonable precautions were to be made to prevent its spread once trachoma was contracted.

To accomplish these objectives, Francis Leupp, who replaced Jones in 1905, proposed converting an off-reservation school "favorably situated as to climate and hygienic conditions" into a sanitarium school for tubercular children. Applying modern medical science in a suitable environment was essential to the care of tubercular children who were otherwise "returned to their homes to die a lingering death, spreading contagion to others." Leupp recommended the sanitarium be constructed at a site in the Southwest, with Phoenix selected as the most suitable location in 1905.[10]

New Health Studies

Leupp was the first commissioner of Indian affairs to tackle the challenges of Indian health care, and once he made the decision to attack tuberculosis, it became foremost on his agenda because of its potential to decimate tribes. He dispatched Elsie E. Newton from the Indian Service to prepare an exhibit for the Sixth Annual Congress on Tuberculosis, meeting in Washington, DC, in 1908, an event at which Leupp admitted tuberculosis "was the greatest single menace to the Indian." Leupp argued the causes of disease were cultural, with communalism and the Indians' superstitious beliefs at the top of his list of causes. These conditions "afforded fruitful soil for the spread of tuberculosis among a people who are exceedingly susceptible to it." The commissioner designated physicians as "health officers" and gave them authority to inspect Indian homes and enforce corrections of unsanitary conditions in an effort to combat disease.[11]

In the months preceding the congress, the Smithsonian Institute detailed Ales Hrdlicka to survey the extent of tuberculosis in Indian Country. Hrdlicka discovered a disparate ratio of Indian men to Indian women, an unusual phenomenon. Among the Menominee, for instance, men outnumbered women 7:6, a phenomenon Hrdlicka attributed to the Menominee accepting remnants of neighboring tribes as members. Without this good neighbor policy, the Menominee would have decreased "as a result of the high mortality largely caused by tuberculosis." Among the Hoopa, the use of a traditional basket bowl passed "freely to well and sick alike" was the prime means of spreading tuberculosis. The tribe had a glandular tuberculosis rate of 193.2 per 1,000 and a pulmonary rate of 60.4 per 1,000.[12] At Phoenix Indian School, twenty-eight Papagos were enrolled in the fall of 1907 after they were found to be in good health. By the following July, five had returned home with symptoms of tuberculosis with two (possibly four) subsequently dying. Such incidents were not unusual: "deadly disease was being spread at the school[s]." The morbidity and mortality rates among the Indians in general far exceeded those among non-Indians and even exceeded the very high rate among blacks.[13]

In 1908, Leupp ordered a special study of Haskell Indian School, a large boarding school in Kansas that educated many of the brightest students in Indian Country. Leupp was stunned by what he discovered. Tuberculosis was not only prevalent among the students but the unsanitary conditions of the school were the causes of contagious diseases. As was too common in Indian schools, dormitories were still overcrowded, poorly lighted and lacked proper ventilation. Students "slept two, three, or more in single beds." Students with pulmonary and glandular tuberculosis "occup[ied] beds with supposedly healthy pupils." Towels and drinking cups were frequently shared and a lack of fresh air "in the dormitories [was] the rule rather than the exception. No attention was paid to decayed teeth and toothbrushes were not regularly used or their use insisted upon. Spitting on the floor was a common occurrence." If conditions such as these existed at Haskell, they were likely far worse at other Indian schools. The Haskell study reinforced the belief that "tuberculosis was spreading rapidly both at home and in these institutions."[14]

The exposure of unhealthy conditions and the prevalence of tuberculosis at Haskell served as the catalyst for a larger campaign against disease. At Haskell, students infected with tuberculosis were immediately sent home (where they may or may not have received care) and all students suspected of having tuberculosis were isolated and monitored. Dorm rooms were to be provided with adequate ventilation and school administrators were forbidden to place more than one student to a bed. New regulations were issued for all schools in the Indian Service.

While acknowledging the "urgent need of doing more than has ever been done before in the way of protecting the Indians against the ravages of the disease," Leupp also conceded the need to protect the non-Indian community. "The infected Indian community becomes a peril to every white community near it," the commissioner commented in 1908. Admitting it was impossible to change the ways of "old-fashioned Indians," Leupp recognized the Indian Service could do more for children. To that end, Leupp established sanitarium camps under the watchful eyes of physicians. Schools disinfected all wind instruments and even fumigated textbooks. The education of Indian children was the key to their survival; it was not to be the cause of their demise.[15]

The Indian Medical Service

The grim conditions convinced Leupp that he had to act and organize an Indian medical service to ensure a minimal level of organization for, and provision of, medical care to the Indians. In conducting the investigation at Haskell, Leupp employed a national tuberculosis expert named Dr. Joseph A. Murphy. Leupp was so impressed with Murphy that he convinced him to stay as the first chief medical supervisor of the Indian Service in 1908.[16] In his new role, Murphy dedicated himself to finding ways to combat tuberculosis and other unsanitary conditions in Indian Country. Addressing the forty-seventh annual gathering of the National Education Association, in 1909, Murphy rhetorically asked if the nation had "not been guilty of criminal negligence" for not doing more to prevent the spread of tuberculosis. The International Congress on Tuberculosis awakened the Indian Service as to the severity of disease. Murphy now encouraged Indian Service teachers, matrons, disciplinarians and superintendents that their duties went further than "the mental welfare of the child." It had to promote their physical welfare as well.[17]

Murphy and a staff of three spent the better part of a year evaluating schools throughout Indian Country, lamenting the policy of sending sick children home from school where more often than not they died. Heeding Murphy's recommendation, Leupp oversaw the construction of screened porches to house tubercular children at a number of Indian school hospitals, a policy Leupp's successor Robert G. Valentine (1909-1912), continued. Tubercular hospital camps were established at Colville, Washington, and Laguna, New Mexico. Sanitarium schools were established in Phoenix, Arizona; Fort Apache, Arizona; Fort Lapwai, Idaho; and Salem, Oregon. An educational campaign designed to foster a better understanding of tuberculosis among school children was also initiated.[18]

The challenges of infectious diseases were so acute that after 1908 every Indian commissioner gave health matters a prominent place in their annual report to Congress. The mortality rate from tuberculosis was 7.71 per thousand (30% of all Indian deaths) in 1909, with the rate rising to 10.4 per thousand (40% of all Indian deaths) the following year. This rate, as Murphy correctly pointed out, was more apparent than real, as statistical errors accounted for much of the increase. Nonetheless, the rate was 60% greater than the prevailing non-Indian rate. An excessive tuberculosis rate among Alaska Natives was called "a needless sacrifice of life." Some of the responsibility for the high rate of disease was credited to the Indians, as many resisted what they perceived as "unwarranted interference" by agency personnel or refused treatment due to cultural taboos. When advice was offered, some simply disregarded or refused it. Even among those who accepted treatment, many failed to follow-through, an issue that Murphy admitted was not unreasonable. If the tables were turned and non-Indians needed assistance, Murphy suggested, they would act similarly.[19]

The Public Health Service Study of 1913

Tuberculosis was the catalyst for creating an Indian medical service. But it was not the only scourge facing American Indians. Trachoma, an eye disease that led to blindness, was also prevalent. The 1903 health survey indicated trachoma (or granulated eyelids) was widespread and caused by environmental factors. Leupp issued yet another circular letter to Indian schools and agencies directing all eye diseases to be treated. To prevent its spread, the commissioner reminded agents trachoma was contagious and the "furnishing of individual towels" was mandatory.[20]

By 1909, trachoma reached a crisis stage, with U.S. Surgeon General Walter Wyman informing Leupp that the increasing prevalence of the disease was "a distinct menace to the public health." The economic self-sufficiency of the Indians—long an Indian Service objective—was endangered with the spread of trachoma, Wyman added, to say nothing of the risks it posed to non-Indians living among and near the Indians. Leupp acted quickly, seeking a special appropriation from Congress to deal with the crisis. In February, Congress agreed to Leupp's request, appropriating $12,000 for trachoma treatment and prevention. With the disease especially rampant among the Indians of the Southwest, a trachoma hospital was opened at Phoenix Indian School and staffed by a trachoma specialist. By 1911, an assistant medical supervisor, a supervisor of field matrons and two other specialists were employed at the new hospital, where 700 cases were treated during the first year.[21]

Two of the specialists in Phoenix visited schools and agencies throughout the Southwest while a third traveled to the Pacific Northwest. Nearly 20,000 Indians were checked for trachoma, with nearly one in five stricken with the disease. Outbreaks of measles were common, particularly in the Southwest. To combat the outbreak, Congress appropriated an additional $40,000 "to relieve distress among the Indians and to provide for their care and for the prevention and treatment of tuberculosis, trachoma, smallpox and other infectious and contagious diseases." With this first-ever general appropriation for Indian health, the Indian Service laid claim to small political gains in the campaign against tuberculosis and trachoma.[22]

In 1915, Congress appropriated $300,000 for Indian health, although critics argued there was scant reason Congress did "not appropriate two to three million dollars a year to put an end to the miseries." Valentine, who replaced Leupp on June 19, 1909, charted a slightly different course of action, stressing the need to combat disease in general, and tuberculosis and trachoma in particular, through education, sanitation inspections and focusing attention on the welfare of children. The methodology inherent in the campaign required a scientific-based program of "modern preventive medicine."[23]

Much was yet unknown about the overall extent of disease among the Indians. Absent a broader understanding of the challenge, progress was difficult. Without a comprehensive investigation to compile a "more accurate registration of vital statistics" and evaluate "contagious and infectious disease," the Indian Service was fettered in its goal of improving health conditions.[24] Although funding increased, the department still had finite resources. Nothing short of an all-out war on disease was warranted. Understaffed and underfunded, the Indian Service did no better than meet emergencies. Valentine had to somehow impress upon Congress the urgency of appropriating funds to make a comprehensive medical survey of Indian Country to determine a benchmark of well-being. Despite insufficient funds, the Indian medical service managed to evaluate 40,000 Indians through a series of isolated surveys by 1912.

Valentine found an ally in President William Howard Taft. On August 10, 1912, Taft delivered a special address to Congress stressing that the "present conditions of health on Indian reservations and in many Indian schools are, broadly speaking, very unsatisfactory." The Indian death rate was more than twice the non-Indian rate (thirty-five versus fifteen deaths per thousand), Taft lamented, and at least 16% of the Indians suffered from trachoma (with 71% of school children from the Kiowa-Comanche-Apache Reservation plagued by the disease). "As guardians of the welfare of the Indians," the President pronounced, "it is our duty to give the race a fair chance for an unmaimed birth, healthy childhood, and a physically efficient maturity."[25]

The President impressed upon Congress the need to increase the annual remuneration of Indian Service physicians, noting, while there were efficient and self sacrificing physicians in the Indian department, "the smallness of the salaries," which averaged $1,186 per year (or less than half that of other government agencies), necessarily affected the qualifications and ability of the physicians employed by the department. More than 160,000 Indians were dependent on federal health care with a corps of 160 physicians, one-third of whom were contract and part-time and most of whom were so scattered that it was common for physicians to drive a day or more to reach isolated families. To this end, Taft recommended the Indian Service "be substantially increased in size" and "lifted into efficiency through the better men whom as a rule only better salaries can command."[26]

Taft asked Congress for a special appropriation of $253,350.[27] He sought $100,000 for a new tuberculosis sanitarium for adults, as there was no such facility for Indians in the United States. He requested $85,000 to increase the salaries of physicians; $1,000 for a pathological laboratory; $10,000 for transportation equipment for physicians and nurses; $2,000 for standard medical literature for physicians; and additional funds for building sleeping porches at boarding schools and hospitals, correcting sanitary deficiencies in Indian homes, providing schools with playground equipment and for producing health literature for distribution to Indian school children. Congress granted him $90,000.

Table 4

Indians Suffering from Trachoma, 1912

State	Number Examined	Percent Trachomatous
Oklahoma	3,252	68.7%
Wyoming	392	51.0%
Nebraska	322	41.0%
Utah	182	39.0%
Iowa	53	32.1%
Virginia	43	30.2%
Nevada	851	26.9%
Montana	2,042	26.3%
Arizona	5,873	24.9%
North Dakota	3,447	22.9%
New Mexico	2,207	22.4%
Kansas	834	21.1%
South Dakota	6,121	17.2%
Idaho	526	16.0%
Colorado	262	15.6%
California	1,555	15.3%
Minnesota	3,542	15.1%
Pennsylvania	552	13.8%
Washington	1,347	13.4%
Oregon	904	10.4%
Michigan	643	7.5%
North Carolina	317	7.0%
Wisconsin	2,999	6.9%
New York	943	0.2%
Florida	22	0.0%
Total (25 States)	39,231	22.7%

(Source: Public Health Service, 1913)

Although the Indian Service did not receive all it requested, the President's message awakened the legislative branch as to the seriousness of ill health in Indian Country. Congress sought a comprehensive evaluation of Indian health but did not trust the Indian Service and instead appropriated $10,000 for the Public Health Service to make a thorough examination "as to the prevalence of tuberculosis, trachoma, smallpox, and other contagious and infectious diseases among the Indians of the United States." In accordance with the Congressional edict, Surgeon General Wyman detailed thirteen medical officers and J.W. Kerr, assistant Surgeon General, to lead the investigation. Kerr began the investigation September 28, 1913, and ended it three months later. Of the 322,715 Indians in the United States, 39,231, or approximately one-eighth of the population, were examined in twenty-five states. The findings of the Public Health Service reinforced what Congress had refrained from accepting: Indian health conditions were not only a menace to non-Indian communities but they were also intolerable. Some 8,940 Indians (23% of the study group) were trachomatous. Extrapolating these numbers over the entire Indian population (excluding Alaska), Kerr conservatively estimated that more than 72,000 Indians suffered from trachoma, with the incidence rate varying from 69% among Oklahoma Indians to 0% among the Indians of Florida, as shown in Table 4.[28]

The prevalence of trachoma in Indian schools was particularly alarming. Of 133 schools visited, 30% of the students (4,916 of 16,470) were trachomatous. At Rainey Mountain (Oklahoma) School, 105 of 114 students (92%) were trachomatous. Only three boarding schools were free of trachoma, one in Wisconsin and two in New York. Kerr legitimized what the Indian Service already knew: trachoma was spread at boarding schools. "Trachoma was found to be generally prevalent in the schools to a greater degree than on the reservations from which the pupils are drawn," the study concluded, "and in non-reservation boarding schools it was found that groups of pupils, from areas where trachoma is absent or but slightly prevalent, presented a high percentage of infection." Kerr conjectured students contracted the disease at the boarding schools "and on their return to their homes they may be the means of implanting a disease in territory where it is now absent or uncommon."[29]

The incidence of the disease in day schools corresponded with the general rate of disease on the reservations, supporting the hypothesis that high rates of trachoma in boarding schools resulted from its spread among the students in such facilities. Half of the trachoma cases involved children between the ages of six and twenty, and it struck girls at a disproportionate rate with boys. Dr. Paul Preble, who examined the Sioux reservations in South Dakota, uncovered one reason for the high rates of disease. Describing a family of eight living and sleeping in a twelve foot by fourteen foot room, Preble was astounded by what he saw: A stove giving off great amounts of heat and foul odor, stifling air, filthy rags and hides. "When an examination of their eyes was attempted," Preble noted, "this mother wiped the discharges from her own eyes with her fingers and then attempted to assist in opening her baby's eyes for examination."[30]

The Public Health Service also provided the first concrete evidence that tuberculosis was not only a menace to Indian health but also increasing in frequency. Its incidence rate ranged from 33% of the Pyramid Lake Paiute to 1% of the Iroquois in New York. As high as the prevalence of tuberculosis was, it was thought to actually be much higher since medical staff could not adequately examine the Indians without bringing them to a clinic. The ubiquitous nature of the disease was "greatly in excess" of that among non-Indians and was "so serious as to require the prosecution of vigorous measures for its relief." Table 5 provides the incidence rate of tuberculosis among the Indians by state. The rate among the white population per thousand was 12.1 and among blacks it was 33.9; for American Indians it was 46.9.[31]

Table 5

Tuberculosis Among the Indians by State, 1912*

State	Examined	Tuberculosis	Incidence Rate**
Iowa	53	8	150.9
Nevada	851	124	145.7
Oregon	1,104	154	139.5
Montana	2,042	247	120.9
Virginia	43	3	69.7
Washington	1,347	73	54.1
Idaho	461	23	49.8
Minnesota	3,542	172	48.5
Pennsylvania	552	26	47.1
Utah	182	8	43.9
North-South Dakota	9,568	361	37.7
Wyoming	392	13	33.1
Wisconsin	2,999	89	29.6
Michigan	643	15	23.3
Arizona	5,873	114	19.4
North Carolina⁴	317	6	18.9
New York	865	11	12.7
Florida	22	0	0.0
Total (19 States)	30,856	1,447	46.9

*California, Colorado, Kansas, Nebraska, New Mexico and Oklahoma unavailable
**per thousand

(Source: Public Health Service, 1913)

The Public Health Service conceded the challenging duties of Indian

Service physicians. Environmental and cultural differences made matters trying. The physical and geographical isolation of reservations and the inadequate financial compensation, absence of promotions and lack of a coordinated medical organization were compounded by the lack of *espirit de corps*. Moreover, physicians lacked substantive authority over medical and sanitary matters in Indian Country.

The Public Health Service study furnished policy-makers a level of reality regarding these challenges. To control the spread of the disease—let alone prevent it—the Surgeon General recommended the Indian Service implement preventive health measures and construct hospitals on all reservations. Transporting patients to off-reservation facilities was ill advised, both to prevent the spread of disease to neighboring communities and to limit the cultural and environmental changes that often compounded disease. To improve home treatment and provide instruction for those without access to hospitals or dispensaries, the Public Health Service recommended the employment of additional nurses.[32]

The causes of unsanitary conditions were well known. Overcrowded homes, uncleanliness and improper diets were the primary causes, although inadequate and unsanitary houses remained a special problem, with the transition from traditional to modern homes proving to be difficult.[33] These sobering conditions were most prevalent on isolated reservations across the West. "Prior to the subjugation of the Indians by white men, they enjoyed an open-air, roving life, living in well-ventilated tepees, which were frequently moved from place to place," Kerr wrote. While unsanitary conditions were "minimized by the frequent moving of camps," confinement to reservations and "more permanent abodes" resulted in an outburst of disease. Many American Indians remained ignorant of the "elementary principles of domestic hygiene and their practical application." It was not unusual for eight or ten people to live in makeshift homes where bedding consisted of "a miscellaneous collection of quilts, blankets and skins, often very filthy." Towels—if available—were shared by all.[34]

These same conditions—overcrowding, poor ventilation and insanitary washing facilities—were still present in boarding schools, institutions used by the Indian Service to accomplish its goal of cultural assimilation. In an Arizona boarding school, 34% of the 249 students leaving the school in the previous ten years died of tuberculosis, although the death rate was probably much higher than reported, as death records were incomplete between 1904 and 1910. Despite departmental circulars of 1904-1905, Indian schools were still operating with inadequate or non-existent medical supervision.

Congress could no longer sit passively. As guardians of the nation's wards, it was forced to reckon with health conditions in Indian Country. With allotment and the sale of surplus lands to non-Indians opening up reservations, lawmakers were compelled to act. That they did so as much to prevent the spread of disease to non-Indians as to ensure the Indians were given a fair chance of success on their own was taken for granted, much to the chagrin of the critics.[35] The $90,000 appropriated for Indian health care in 1913 was more than doubled to $200,000 the following year. In 1914, Congress appropriated $100,000 for the construction of hospitals among the Blackfeet, Turtle Mountain Chippewa, Mescalero Apache, Gila River Pima, San Xavier Papago and the scattered Indians near Carson, Nevada. An additional $10,000 was set aside to equip the old Fort Spokane military reservation with an Indian hospital.[36]

Save the Children

With additional funds, Murphy and Indian Commissioner Cato Sells (who replaced Valentine in 1913) launched a campaign to improve Indian health care. The number of hospitals, which stood at fifty-three in 1913, nearly doubled by 1920. While most were small and inadequately staffed, they marked a new beginning in the war on disease. In an effort to foil the spread of trachoma, the Indian Service established five medical districts in Indian Country with an ophthalmologist assigned to each to instruct reservation physicians on appropriate methods of eye care. The ophthalmologist handled serious eye complications requiring special treatment or surgery and supported local physicians through training. Heeding the advice of Murphy, Sells ordered individual Pullman towels installed in all Indian schools beginning in 1914. Combined with the segregation of acute trachomatous students and the implementation of regular eye treatments, trachoma was mitigated for the first time in some Indian schools. Five dentists were also assigned to the medical branch in 1914, devoting their time to the dental needs of a small number of boarding school children and, when time permitted, for a limited number of adults.[37]

Beyond the campaign against tuberculosis and trachoma, the focus of Sells' agenda was reducing infant mortality. To deal with the challenge, Sells continued a program initiated by Valentine called "Save the Babies." Increasing awareness of the causes of infant mortality was important to the overall improvement of health conditions. "It is our duty to protect the Indian's health and to save him from premature death," Sells stated in an opening address before the Congress on Indian Progress. "Before we educate him, before we conserve his property, we should save his life. If he is to be perpetuated, we must care for the children. We must stop the tendency of the Indian to diminish in number, and restore a condition that will ensure his increase." To do this, Indian hospital beds not utilized were made available for childbirth. It was the children, Sells stressed, who were of prime importance in reestablishing the health of the Indians. Everything—including property and education—was "secondary to the basic condition that makes for the perpetuation of the race."[38]

In a circular letter addressed to Indian Service employees, the Commissioner outlined the fundamental challenge. "No race," Sells explained, "was ever created for utter extinction." In 1916, he asked employees to develop "a righteous passion to see that every Indian child has a fair chance to live." The Indian problem could not be solved without Indians and Indians could not be educated unless they were kept alive. The goal of federal-Indian policy was the perpetuation of "an enduring and sturdy race." That could only begin with the children. To correspond with the campaign, Sells introduced the "Swat the Fly" campaign to eliminate a prime carrier of disease. More regulations were issued to make privies fly-proof and to insure trash containers were sanitary.[39]

With six of ten Indian children dying prior to their fifth birthday, Sells asked, "Of what use to this mournful mortality are our splendidly equipped schools?" Reservation superintendents were to acquaint themselves with the home conditions of every family. Field matrons encouraged prospective mothers to give birth in hospitals, while physicians insured proper pre- and postnatal care. All employees were instructed to do their part in seeing that children were furnished with proper nourishment. A vigilant staff at the local level, Sells argued, would insure children were afforded every opportunity at a healthy life.

Sells recognized there would be cultural challenges with the Save the Babies campaign but he expected employees to redouble their energy and zeal, "for it means personal work and tireless patience." Sells instituted a series of addresses on child welfare topics for Indian women led by physicians, nurses and matrons. Schools formed little mother leagues to teach older girls about nursing, hygiene, sanitation and caring for children, something Sells saw as "promptly and greatly" profiting young women when they returned to their homes to raise a sibling or have children of their own. Some schools, such as Carlisle, printed material to educate youth. In 1917, Dr. Charles Zimmerman penned "An Appeal for Pre-Natal Care," in *The Red Man*, a publication of Carlisle Indian School. Designed to correspond with the Save the Babies campaign, the appeal urged Indian mothers (or mothers-to-be) to accept pre-natal care to improve the survival rate of their babies.[40]

Accompanying the campaign was a baby contest in which mothers exhibited their healthy babies at Indian fairs held each fall throughout Indian Country. Physicians evaluated the health and well-being of babies, with certificates issued to the parents of the babies scoring the highest. Childcare exhibits and pamphlets—one entitled "Indian Mothers, Save Your Babies"—were distributed as well. The number of infant deaths generally decreased after 1914, leading Sells to boast the American Indians were no longer a vanishing race. Despite a drop in the infant mortality rate, infant diseases remained high among Indians, as shown in Table 6.[41]

The campaign against disease made headway in part due to the first specific Indian health appropriations. American entry into World War One, however, interrupted this campaign and, in some areas, brought it to a halt. The war effort devastated the Indian Service, with 40% of the physician posts vacant. One out of seven contract physician posts was vacant as were forty-four of the ninety-nine nursing positions. Postwar inflation and a reduction in Indian health expenditures crippled long-term advancements in the campaign against infant mortality and disease.

Table 6

Infant Mortality Among American Indians: 1914-1920

Year	Births	Deaths	Under Three	Percent Under 3
1914	6,964	5,778	2,391	41%
1915	6,542	5,632	1,897	33%
1916	6,092	4,570	1,303	28%
1917	5,340	4,494	1,379	30%
1918	5,571	4,682	1,541	32%
1919	6,344	*9,462	1,644	17%
1920	6,510	6,070	1,436	23%
Totals	42,868	40,788	11,591	28%

*Increase due to outbreak of influenza in 1918-1919

(Source: *Tuberculosis Among the North American Indians*, 1921)

If World War One alone had interrupted the campaign against disease it would have been devastating enough. Added to the wartime reductions was the world-wide outbreak of Spanish influenza in 1918, which struck especially hard in Indian Country. Out of a population of 304,854, there were 73,651 cases of influenza among American Indians, with 6,270 succumbing to the disease. More than 2% of the American Indians died, versus .6% of all Americans.[42] The combination of war-time vacancies and influenza did more than cut short progress in Indian Country; it left critical work unattended. Every trachoma specialist in the Indian Service was reassigned during the epidemic, with all trachoma work abandoned.

Economy and Renewed Criticism

The election of 1920 brought a Republican-led downsizing of the federal government. Economy was the new buzzword, with Indian policy seeking to emancipate the Indians from government supervision and responsibility. The Indian Service was targeted for budget reductions and even discussions of elimination. Reformers of the day viewed the government as "hopelessly stagnant and even venal." While critics blamed the Indian Service for the deplorable conditions in Indian Country, they rarely considered the federal office was simply the appointed tool for carrying out Congressional intent. "[M]aking bricks without straw has limits," one Indian Service employee complained, reminding readers that Congress controlled the purse of the Indian Service.[43]

Commissioner of Indian Affairs Charles Burke (1921-1929) followed the legislative lead of Congress and enforced economy within the agency. The result was hardly unexpected: the Indian medical service came under renewed scrutiny. The specious assumptions of the old assimilationists, who believed the Indians were biologically and/or culturally inferior to non-Indians, were replaced in the 1920s when a new series of studies indicated the Indians were diseased not because of genetic deficiencies but because of environmental conditions in Indian Country. Since it was the Indian Service that was responsible for carrying out the whims of Congress, it bore the brunt of the criticism, even though a parsimonious Congress turned a deaf ear to the needs of the Indians.

The Indian Service also came under intense scrutiny from members of the American Medical Association. Dr. Otis O. Benson, for instance, a former Indian Service physician and superintendent, declared "open season" on the department. Citing a litany of common criticisms, including inadequate pay, lack of basic equipment, muddled channels of communication, Indian resistance and Congressional apathy, Benson informed the American Medical Association of the poor success of the Indian medical service. Other critics, such as Frederick L. Hoffman, were less kind. "There is," Hoffman opined, "broadly speaking, no Indian health service, and very little is done to prevent occurrences of disease."[44]

Burke, asked to do more with less, responded to the criticisms in 1922 by asking Judge John Barton Payne, Chairman of the American Red Cross, to conduct a survey to determine the need for public health nurses in Indian Country. Payne appointed Florence M. Patterson, a fifteen-year public health veteran, hospital administrator, and graduate of Northwestern University and John Hopkins Training School for Nurses, to lead the investigation. Patterson spent nine months traveling across Indian Country in Arizona, New Mexico, California and Utah. What she uncovered would have shocked the nation—if Burke had allowed her report to be made public.[45]

Patterson's report made the most vociferous critics of the Indian Service appear benign. While blurring the line between actual conditions and what could be done with public health nurses, Patterson condemned nearly every aspect of the Indian medical service. Reservation vital statistics, Patterson noted, were frequently copied from year to year "with slight variations." If an agency had no medical staff, employees simply made educated guesses to fill in medical records. One agency failed to record any causes of death. The superintendent informed Patterson he could recall the causes of death for those who died without medical care. "This boy died in February," the superintendent explained, and "undoubtedly it was pneumonia." When a baby died, the same superintendent stated, "This baby's mother had tuberculosis; therefore, in all probability he died of it, too."[46]

Despite fragmentary and erroneous statistics, Patterson conceded that conditions described by critics represented a credible view of reservation life. Even though the Indian birth rate was 26% higher than the national average, the death rate was 163% higher, painting a picture of needless suffering and despair. With the Indian birth rate at 30.4 per thousand and the death rate of 30.5 per thousand (compared to comparable non-Indian rates of 24.3 and 11.7, respectively), the Indians' chance of survival was precarious at best. Tuberculosis was six times greater than the non-Indian rate and, as others reported earlier, boarding schools "frequently facilitated, rather than prevented" disease. One sixteen-year-old girl, without warning or suspicion of tuberculosis, had a "profuse pulmonary hemorrhage." After thirty-six hours in the school hospital, she was discharged and told to return to school, only to have another hemorrhage while standing in the doorway. That night she had a third hemorrhage. Two days later she was sent home, with both the school doctor and nurse believing their responsibility ended there.[47]

Trachoma was irregularly examined and then only when an eye specialist visited a reservation. Often times, boarding school teachers were required to administer treatment to trachomatous students. Anywhere from 40% to 75% of the school children were infected with trachoma. At the Pima boarding school, the rate was 50%, while at Pima day school it was 75%. The rate at nearby Phoenix Indian School was 25%, all lending credence to reports indicating that schools were a source of disease. Patterson blamed the high rates of trachoma and other diseases on the "exacting routine" of the schools, with their strict emphasis on military order. Improper diets compounded matters. A typical breakfast at one school was bread, coffee and syrup, while dinner and supper consisted of bread and boiled potatoes. One vocal critic argued children "sing health poems to milk but receive none." At the same time, children recite "the danger of coffee to childhood and get it three times a day." Notwithstanding departmental circulars, Patterson found overcrowding the norm rather than the exception.[48]

Table 7

Infant Mortality Rates in the Southwest, 1921

Tribe	Deaths per thousand
Hopi	196
Pima	256
Yuma	269
Northern Pueblos	278
Urban South Carolina*	105

*highest incidence rate in the U.S.
(Source: American Red Cross, 1922)

Measles was acute in the Southwest, particularly among the Pima and Papago. While Patterson placed much of the blame on ignorance (i.e., improper diets and lack of understanding causes of disease), environmental factors (poverty and filth) also contributed. Measles added to the "abnormally high infant mortality rate," as shown in Table 7.[49]

If the prevalence of disease didn't indict the Indian Service its administrative structure did. While there were good employees, many physicians and nurses had been rejected by other federal agencies. When competent medical staff was found, they were stymied by the dictatorial control of some agency superintendents. Patterson was not alone in condemning this authority. Elinor Gregg, the first public health nurse in the Indian Service, referred to some superintendencies as "totalitarian states" run by czars, whose "judgment was law." Such czar-like superintendents prevented enforcement of hygienic regulations, sanitation and other health matters—frequently for political reasons but more often because they were "entirely ignorant of modern public health work."[50]

Another challenge to maintaining good health care was nepotism. One competent nurse who knew all of the school children and who had made a significant impact on their welfare was transferred so that another employee's wife could have the position. The new nurse had no contact whatsoever with Indian families. On most reservations in the Southwest, Patterson complained, physicians made calls only when requested. Field matrons had no business in the Indian Service and were, in Patterson's mind, positions to subsidize another agency employee's salary rather than a real job.[51]

Burke was incensed with the report and had it ensconced from official public record, although rumors abounded. Not to be chastised without comment, Burke ordered medical director Robert E. Lee Newberne, who replaced Murphy as medical supervisor in November of 1918, to prepare an analysis of the report. In his rebuttal, Newberne downplayed the role of public health nurses, arguing that if Patterson wanted to undertake greater responsibility she should "take the medical course." He also charged Patterson with trying to present public health nursing "in the best light possible" for personal gain. Reminding Burke—who favored public health nurses—the work of nurses was to care for patient needs "under a physician," not to assume the position of "primary responsibility," Newberne suggested nurses did ordinary service that did not require a high school education. While Patterson elevated nurses, Newberne degraded them. That his motives were political is clear. Public health nurses would be paid out of the limited Indian medical service budget. Field matrons, whom Newberne preferred, were paid out of an Industrial Work and Care of Timber fund that did not impact his budget.[52]

Burke, originally hoping to use a persuasive report to leverage funds from Congress, never submitted the report and prevented any outside agency from reviewing it. When Assistant Commissioner Edgar B. Meritt was asked by the California State Board of Health for a copy, in 1926, he declined. "If your Congressman wants to see the Grace (sic) Patterson report he can come down and see it," Meritt informed the board, "but I doubt very much if the Commissioner of

Indian Affairs would send that report out to an organization to be published." Meritt disputed the conditions described by the Red Cross. Burke officially classified the report as "impractical," fearing more fuel for the fodder for Indian critics—including a newcomer named John Collier. By burying the report, Burke put the Red Cross in the awkward position of having to defend itself. When the Red Cross asked Burke to publish at least part of the report so the organization could discuss the criticisms openly, Burke simply ignored it.[53]

While Burke successfully withheld the Red Cross study from the public, he was powerless to stop a similar—albeit less critical—report made by the National Tuberculosis Association. Entitled *Tuberculosis among the North American Indians*, the study corroborated a growing body of evidence that Indians were not predisposed to tuberculosis as much as their socio-environmental conditions added to their greater likelihood of contracting the disease. While not new, the report documented the frequency of Indian students acquiring tuberculosis while at school. "We find more and more," the California Bureau of Tuberculosis reported, "that the younger Indians, particularly those who have attended the Indian schools, seem to acquire tuberculosis after they leave home to attend school." The transition from a state of outdoor living to an indoor one once again was viewed as a significant cause of the high incidence rate of tuberculosis. To palliate these socio-environmental challenges, the National Tuberculosis Association encouraged Burke to construct two or three additional sanitaria. Despite the continued opposition of Newberne to public health nurses, the Association strongly recommended their employment in Indian Country, something Burke agreed to when he appointed a Red Cross public health nurse named Elinor Gregg to establish demonstration public health projects on the Pine Ridge and Rosebud (South Dakota) Sioux reservations. Augustine B. Stoll was also appointed as public health nurse to the Jicarilla (New Mexico) Apache Reservation. Between them, Gregg and Stoll were to demonstrate the feasibility of operating a public health program in Indian Country, a difficult task considering Newberne opposed their actions.[54]

While the National Tuberculosis Association report was largely a reiteration of earlier surveys and studies, it reinforced the need of the Indian Service—and Congress as guardian—to do more in conserving the health of the Indians. The long-desired assimilation of the Indians envisioned by nineteenth century humanitarians and policy-makers had not occurred, in part, due to the poor health of the Indians. Land severalty presumed individual landowning Indians would be self-supporting, healthy citizens. The reality was far from this. American Indians were in a state of severe economic and social deprivation. Environmental challenges combined with the continued rapid push for cultural absorption, manifested themselves in a distraught, deteriorated and diseased people. There was no greater disappointment than in the conditions of the Indian schools. The Indian Service was vulnerable to criticism. A new choral of critics was "bent on proving that the Indian Service was either stupid or venal, or both." So severe was the criticism, that Congress considered transferring the Indian medical service into the Public Health Service.[55]

Notes

1. Warren K. Moorehead, *The American Indians in the United States: 1850-1914* (Freeport, New York: Books for Liberty Press, 1969 reprint edition of the 1914 original), 265; Haven Emerson, "Morbidity of the American Indians," *Science* (68:1626, February 26, 1926), 230.

2. Thornton, 101, argued, "because of vaccinations late 19th century American Indians felt the effects of smallpox less than adjacent populations of non-Indians." Most outbreaks after 1890 were localized. Education Circular no. 31, August 5, 1899, RG, M1121, *Office of Indian Affairs, Circulars*, roll 8.

3. L. Webster Fox, "Conditions in the Indian Medical Service," *Journal of the American Medical Association*, November 3, 1923, 1574; The Indian Service "historical review" is found in *The Indian Service Health Activities* (1922). Lummis to Moorehead, in Moorehead, 267. Thirty years prior tuberculosis was "almost unknown" in the Pueblos of New Mexico, Lummis wrote, and "the first consumptive Pueblo I ever saw was from Carlisle [Indian School]." Frederick L. Hoffman, "Conditions in the Indian Service," *Journal of the American Medical Association*, (75:7, August 14, 1920), 493.

4. Washington Matthews, "Consumption Among the Indians," *Transactions of the American Climatological Association*, 1886, 234-241. Matthews, "Further Contribution to the Study of Consumption Among the Indians," ibid, 136-155. McConnell to Hitchcock, July 29, 1899. RG 48, *Letters Received, Office of Indian Affairs*, Official Letters of W. J. McConnell, U.S. Indian Inspector.

5. McConnell to Hitchcock, June 17, 1901, RG 48, *Letters Received, Office of the Secretary of Interior*, Indian Division, Indian Inspection Reports, Blackfeet. McConnell to Hitchcock, July 5, 1901; RG 48, *Letters Received, Office of the Secretary of the Interior*, Appointments Division, Indian Inspectors, W. J. McConnell. "Conditions of Reservation Indians, Letter from the Secretary of the Interior," dated February 21, 1901, *House Document no. 406*, 57th Congress, 1st Session (Washington, DC: GPO, 1901), 26.

6. *Annual Report*, "Report of the Superintendent of Indian Schools," 1898, 340-341. It was difficult for the Indian Service to adapt its focus from a strict bureaucratic system of decision-making and share power with physicians. Lack of support for developing a civil service exam compounded the matter.

7. Education Circular no. 102, September 21, 1903. Circular no. 85, dated November 6, 1902, directed off-reservation schools to admit only "sound and healthy children." A physician's certificate was to accompany each student before he could be admitted to school. RG 75, M1121, *Office of Indian Affairs, Circulars*, roll 9.

8. *Regulations for the Indian Department*, (Washington, DC: GPO, 1884), 97-99. *Annual Report*, 1894, 89-92; *Annual Report*, 1904, 33-38.

9. *Annual Report*, 1904, 33-38. Despite new circulars from the commissioner in 1903 and 1904, it was not until 1906 that the directives were implemented by the agencies.

10. Francis E. Leupp, "Outlines of an Indian Policy," *Outlook* (79, April 15,

1905), 946-950. *Annual Report*, 1905, 1-15. The first students were placed in the East Farm Sanatorium at Phoenix Indian School in May of 1909. Robert A. Trennert Jr., *The Phoenix Indian School: Forced Assimilation in the Desert, 1891-1935* (Norman: University of Oklahoma Press, 1988), 105. There were thirty-nine students admitted the first year. The facility was located 1 ¼ miles east of Phoenix Indian School on the school farm. Dr. Jacob Breid, writing in 1914, acknowledged that before the sanatorium opened students were often sent home without care. Breid, "East Farm Sanatorium School," *The Red Man*, 6:9, May 1914 (Carlisle Indian School Publication), 362-367. By 1913, of the 220 students passing through the facility, fifty-two had their tuberculosis arrested, 109 showed improvement, twenty-three showed no improvement, thirty-one died, and five were unknown.

11. *Transactions of the Sixth International Congress on Tuberculosis*, six volumes (Philadelphia: William F. Fall, 1908) vol. 4, part 1, 428-435.

12. Ales Hrdlicka, "Tuberculosis among Certain Indian Tribes in the United States," *Bureau of American Ethnology Bulletin 42* (Washington, DC: Government Printing Office, 1909), 4.

13. Francis Paul Prucha, *The Great Father: The United States Government and the American Indians*, Volume II (Lincoln: University of Nebraska Press, 1984), 847. Hrdlicka visited the Menominee, Oglala Sioux, Quinaielt, Hoopa and Mojave, in addition to Phoenix Indian School. All of the Hoopa and Mojave were evaluated and 100 families from the Oglala Sioux and Menominee were screened. Only full-blooded Oglalas were checked. Hrdlicka, "Tuberculosis among Certain Indian Tribes of the United States," 8, 17, 25 and 26. "Fighting the White Plague," *Annual Report*, 1908, 24. Trennert, 103.

14. *Tuberculosis among the North American Indians*, 97.

15. Leupp, "Fighting the White Plague," *Annual Report*, 1908, 23-24.

16. Murphy received a special appointment as medical supervisor on November 23, 1908, without having to go through the usual civil service exam. Leupp appointed Murphy temporarily as "an emergency matter." Temporary appointments could not exceed three months, so Murphy was reappointed three times before being appointed permanently on January 5, 1910. This was after the Indian Service helped the civil service create an appropriate civil service exam for the position. Murphy's score was only the second highest (84.75%), behind Ferdinand Shoemaker of Oklahoma (91.45%). At Valentine's request, Murphy was appointed. "Report in the Matter of the Investigation of the Indian Bureau with transcripts of Testimony Taken and Exhibits Offered from April 9, 1912 to August 17, 1912," *House Report no. 1279*, (Washington, DC: GPO, 1913), 62nd Congress, 3rd session, 198-205.

17. Joseph F. Murphy, "The Prevention of Tuberculosis in the Indian Schools," *Journal of Proceedings and Addresses of the Forty-Seventh Annual Meeting*, (Winona, Minnesota: National Education Association, Secretary's Office, 1909), 919-924. Murphy lamented the tendency of the schools to "handle the mass rather the individual," a practice that frequently neglected Indian welfare.

18. Murphy, *Manual on Tuberculosis: Its Causes, Prevention, and Treatment*, (Washington, DC: GPO, 1910). Valentine, in the 1909 *Annual Report* (5-6), outlined the following line of attack. Better nourishment; improved sanitary conditions; complete sterilization of dishes; revised methods of sweeping and dusting; fumigation of all schools and books; establishment of a traveling health exhibit; a course on physical development

and health care; distribution of a pamphlet on tuberculosis prevention and cure; establishment of tuberculosis camps; and more sanitary homes for Indians with proper ventilation.

19. Murphy, "Health Problems of the Indians," *The Annals of the American Academy of Political and Social Science* (Philadelphia, 37:2, March 1911), 347-353. In April 1908, the House of Representatives indicated that the problem of tuberculosis was not confined just to the continental United States. A report from Captain Paul C. Hutton, Assistant Surgeon, U.S. Army, Fort William Seward, Alaska Territory, dated October 28, 1907, points out that nearly half of the Alaska Native population in his district was affected with tuberculosis. "Report of Captain Paul C. Hutton, Assistant Surgeon, U.S. Army, Office of the Surgeon, Fort William Seward, October 28, 1907, to the Adjutant-General, Department of the Columbia, Vancouver Barracks, Washington," in *House Report No. 1372*, "To Provide for Compulsory Education of Native Children of Alaska, and for the Enforcement of Sanitary Regulations among the Natives of Alaska," April 2, 1908, 60th Congress, 1st session, (Washington, DC: GPO, 1909), 3-5.

20. *Annual Report*, 1904, 36. It was not until 1901 that any meaningful attention was given by the Indian Service to the treatment of trachoma and then only after an outbreak of trachoma at Phoenix Indian School. Trennert, 76-77, notes a measles epidemic in December 1899 brought 325 cases of the disease along with sixty cases of pneumonia.

21. "An Act for the Investigation, Treatment, and Prevention of Trachoma among the Indians," 35 stat. 642. "Trachoma in Certain Indian Schools," *Senate Report No. 1025*, 60th Congress, 2nd session, (Washington, DC: GPO, 1909), 2.

22. 32 Stat. 271. In 1912 the appropriation increased to $60,000 and in 1913 it jumped to $90,000.

23. *Annual Report*, 1910, 9-10. Not everyone was satisfied with the appropriations. Moorehead, 267, opined, "there is no earthly excuse why instead of three or four, there should not be fifteen or twenty doctors on every reservation."

24. Murphy, "Health Problems of the Indians," 103-104.

25. William Howard Taft, "Diseases among the Indians: Message from the President of the United States in Relation to the Present Conditions of Health on Indian Reservations and in Indian Schools," August 10, 1912, *Senate Document no. 907*, 62nd Congress, 2nd session, (Washington, DC: GPO, 1912), 1-3.

26. *Senate Document no. 907*. Change would be along "carefully planned business lines and without extravagance, and after a comparative study other medical services, National, State and local."

27. *Annual Report*, 1912, 17-22. The appropriation request is found in "Diseases among the Indians: A Letter from the Acting Secretary of the Treasury transmitting a copy of a Letter from the Secretary of the Interior, August 14, 1912," *Senate Document no. 920*, 62nd Congress, 2nd session, (Washington, DC: GPO, 1912). In writing Acting Secretary James F. Curtis, Interior Secretary Walter L. Fisher outlined the appropriation needs and the comparative salaries. Indian Service medical supervisors ($3,000) made fifty percent of that paid to Navy, Army and Public Health Service directors. Indian Service assistant medical directors made less than fifty percent ($2,200 versus $5,000) and Indian Service physicians were paid, on average, $900 to $1,400 per

annum versus $2,000 to $2,640 for other government physicians.

28. 37 Stat. 519.

29. "Contagious and Infectious Diseases among the Indians," *Senate Document no. 1038*, 62nd Congress, 3rd session, (Washington, DC: GPO, 1913), 74.

30. "Contagious and Infectious Diseases among the Indians," 62-63.

31. "Contagious and Infectious Diseases among the Indians," 77.

32. "Contagious and Infectious Diseases among the Indians," 82-84.

33. Valentine, in 1912, issued a special circular entitled "Our Task." In it he stressed no stone was to be left unturned in getting every Indian family a sanitary house. Every effort was to be made to "reduce infant mortality. Save the Babies" was to be the primary objective. In schools, diseased children were to be segregated "no matter at what loss to scholastic achievement." Circular no. 633, April 29, 1912, RG 75, M1121, *Office of Indian Affairs, Circulars*, roll 10.

34. "Contagious and Infectious Diseases among the Indians," 61-63.

35. *Annual Report*, 1914, 14. Moorehead, 273, wrote that when non-Indians living in Indian Country cried "menace to public health" Congress acted. But when "Indians complained we pay little heed."

36. Plans were also made to build hospitals on the Red Lake Chippewa and Fond du Lac Chippewa reservations in Minnesota, and within the Choctaw Nation, Oklahoma (to be built using Choctaw-Chickasaw tribal funds). "Letter from the Secretary of the Interior (Franklin Lane) to the House Committee on Indian Affairs," *House Document no. 1254*, 63rd Congress, 2nd session, (Washington, DC: GPO, 1915), 1-2. The appropriation was provided for in the 1915 Indian Appropriation Act, 38 Stat. 582.

37. The fifty-three hospitals were apportioned as follows: Arizona had thirteen; New Mexico, Oklahoma, South Dakota and Wisconsin each had four; California, Idaho, Minnesota and Washington each had three; Montana, Nevada and North Dakota each had two; and Kansas, Michigan, Nebraska, Oregon, Pennsylvania and Wyoming each had one. The average bed size was fewer than 24. "Report of the Joint Commission on Indian Tuberculosis Sanitarium and Yakima Indian Reservation Project," *House Document no. 505*, 63rd Congress, 2nd session, (Washington, DC: GPO, 1912), exhibit C, 19-20. Of the 2,190 beds available, 528 were in off-reservation school hospitals, ninety-two were in the Canton Insane Asylum, 573 were in tuberculosis sanatorium, leaving fewer than 1,000 beds in fifty-seven hospitals in Indian Country. "The Indian Problem: Resolution of the Committee of One Hundred appointed by the Secretary of the Interior and a Review of the Indian Problem," *House Document no. 149*, 68th Congress, 1st Session (Washington, DC: GPO, 1924), 35.

38. *Annual Report*, 1916, 4

39. Circular no. 707, (November 9, 1912 and supplemented January 6, 1914); Circular no. 1263, (February 15, 1917); Circular no. 764 (July 31, 1913); Circular no. 865 (May 20, 1914); Circular no. 933 (June 9, 1915); Circular no. 1003 (July 10, 1915), RG 75, M1121, *Office of Indian Affairs, Circulars*, rolls 10-11.

40. Charles L. Zimmerman, "An Appeal for Prenatal Care," *The Red Man*, 9:7, May-June 1917, 237. Elsie E. Newton, "The Going Home Woman," ibid, 6:9, 374-376.

41. *Annual Report*, 1916, 7. *Annual Report*, 1917, 19. Ales Hrdlicka, "The Vanishing Indian," *Science* (46:1185, September 14, 1917), 266-267.

42. "Influenza among American Indians," *Public Health Reports* 34 (May 9, 1919), 1008-1009.

43. Elinor D. Gregg, *The Indian and the Nurse* (Norman: University of Oklahoma Press, 1965), 71, blamed the Indian Service, suggesting that it "set down the policies" for the medical care of Indians.

44. Otis O. Benson, M.D., "Conditions in the Indian Medical Service," *Journal of the American Medical Association* (81:16, October 20, 1923), 1381-1382. Benson noted Congress scowled at adequate appropriations for the Indian Service. Hoffman, "Conditions in the Indian Medical Service," 493-494. Hoffman urged the transfer of the Indian medical service to the Public Health Service.

45. Patterson visited the Jicarilla, San Carlos and Mescalero Apaches, the Pueblos, the Gila River Pima, the Papago (Sells), Hopi, Western Navajo, Yumas, Ute and Mission Indians of California—in all thirteen agencies. Testimony of Florence M. Patterson, Wednesday, December 12, 1928, in *Survey of Conditions of the Indians in the United States: Hearing Before a Subcommittee of the Committee on Indian Affairs United States Senate*, Part 3 (Washington, DC: GPO, 1929), 933-1018.

46. "A Study of the Need for Public-Health Nursing on Indian Reservations," in ibid, 957.

47. "A Study of the Need for Public-Health Nursing on Indian Reservations," 959, 966, 968. This particular school had physically examined the 137 students enrolled and found none—including this sixteen-year-old girl—infected with tuberculosis.

48. "A Study of the Need for Public-Health Nursing on Indian Reservations," 970.

49. One mother of nine told of losing four children to measles during one epidemic. Patterson wrote that just one agency recorded its infant mortality rate in the Commissioner's annual report. Emerson, 230, noted a limited quantity of milk was provided daily. One little girl, when asked who received the milk, replied, "Oh, the big boys." One cup of milk was typically provided to one-quarter of the students at each meal, or one-fourth of a cup per pupil.

50. One doctor had been discharged from one federal medical service for "reasons which made him unsuitable for any type of medical service," yet he was accepted by the Indian Service. Nursing requirements in the Indian Service ranged from "no training or preparation whatsoever to what is considered an adequate training for hospital service." Salaries remained "incredibly low." (p. 982). Gregg, 12 and 115.

51. "A Study of the Need for Public Health Nursing on Indian Reservations," 984-991, critiques the matrons. Patterson recommended the elimination of field matrons or, at a minimum, placing them under the authority of the director of nursing services (1005).

52. Newberne's rebuttal, "A Review of Miss Patterson's Report entitled 'A Study of the Need for Public Health Nursing on Indian Reservations'," is printed in the *Survey of Conditions of the Indians in the United States*, 1005-1017. Gregg, 80, wrote Newberne "was dead set against the Commissioner's plan of having public-health nurses replace his field matrons."

53. The Red Cross received no reply despite sending two letters to Burke, the first dated January 26, 1927, and the second dated February 11, 1927. "A Study of the

Need for Public Health Nursing on Indian Reservations," 949-950.
   54. *Tuberculosis among the North American Indians*, 29, 45-46. Gregg's effectiveness was severely limited by physicians and superintendents who did not appreciate and value the need for public health measures in Indian Country.
   55. Gregg, 92.

CHAPTER THREE

Reform and Reorganization

By the 1920s, the status of Indian health was at least two generations behind the national average. The American Red Cross and the National Tuberculosis Association reminded the Indian Service of this reality. Taken together, these studies begged the question of whether Congress, as guardians of the nation's wards, had the responsibility to act and whether the nation had a moral obligation to assist the Indians? In the years following First World War, a new generation of Indian reformers answered these questions in the affirmative. Among these reformers that focused on the many positive characteristics of the Indians was an outspoken critic named John Collier. Collier argued culture was as valuable as economics. With the Indian Service focused on economic integration, Collier believed the government's approach to be misguided. Not only was it neglecting its fiduciary responsibility, but it also seemed to be preventing Indians from attaining a state of relatively good health.[1]

While preventive medicine was becoming the norm across the United States, it was slow to materialize in Indian Country, where the emphasis remained curative. Consequently, a sizeable portion of the annual Congressional appropriations went for hospital construction to reduce the backlog of unmet Indian health needs. Although hospitals were an important part of the campaign against disease, they simply handled daily emergencies. Although there were eighty-seven hospitals by 1924, there were still too few facilities, too much inadequate equipment and a too limited and under-trained medical staff to handle the volume of need in Indian Country.

Transfer to the Public Health Service?

The 1920s were a time of important microscopic change in the administration of Indian affairs that cumulatively resulted in a complete departure from the old assimilationist policies of the previous half century. A series of reforms ended the allotment of Indian land, encouraged Indian land consolidation, improved educational resources and brought the first steps in revitalizing tribal governments. Policy changes also impacted Indian health care and services. In this backdrop, social and political critics recommended Congress immediately transfer the Indian health program out of the Indian Service and into the Public Health Service where professionalism was high, funding was adequate and modern science utilized. Looking for ways to economize government activities and spending, the House Committee on Indian Affairs opened hearings on the proposed transfer in September 1919. An increasingly conservative political climate advocated the complete abolition of the Indian Service and the withdrawal of the government from the Indian business. Only by integrating the Indian medical service with the Public Health Service, conventional wisdom opined, could efficiency be attained and the first steps in the final assimilation of the Indians accomplished.[2]

While Congress was keen on the idea of consolidation, neither the Indian Service nor the Public Health Service favored or endorsed such a plan. Surgeon General Robert Blue, while acknowledging such a transfer should eventually occur, opposed consolidation on the grounds that it would be difficult to secure competent physicians to fill the needs of the Indian medical service. Of greater concern was the isolation of most reservations, particularly in the West. Blue did not wish to inherit what he viewed as a political liability and a logistical nightmare. A more immediate political consideration for Blue was the medical care of returning World War One veterans. American servicemen were overwhelming the Public Health Service and, as enfranchised citizens, were of "more importance." Congressman Carl Hayden (D-AZ), a member of the Committee on Indian Affairs, emphasized nothing should disturb the Public Health Service in caring for the troops. The Indian medical service was doing all it could, Blue testified. Clinging to old arguments of cultural inferiority, Blue placed culpability for the high incidence of disease in Indian Country on the strange practices and habits of the Indians.[3]

The Indian Service also opposed any discussion of consolidation. Medical Director Newberne, recognizing it "would be pleasing" to be associated with the Public Health Service, argued health care was too closely allied with the educational and social goals of the Indian Service to warrant such action. Unless Congress was prepared to turn the whole department over to the Public Health Service, Newberne opined, the move was ill advised. Commissioner of Indian Affairs Cato Sells concurred, suggesting that any talk of consolidation was a "radical variance" with standard administrative practices. If the Public Health Service were to assume responsibility for Indian health, Sells opined, it would do no better than the Indian medical service unless "additional appropriations were made." The bottom line, the commissioner boasted, was that the Indians were in a "critical transformation period" of evolving from one "social plain to another" and only the Indian Service was equipped to manage this transformation.[4]

The medical establishment did not waver in its desire to effect the transfer. Frederick Hoffman, statistician for the Prudential Insurance Company and a member of the American Medical Association, argued the transfer called for "the highest considerations of Indian policy" because there was "no health service worthy of the name" in Indian Country. Hoffman was notorious in his critique of the Indian medical service, calling it "as deplorable as it was disgraceful" and "the most regrettable apathy on the part of the nation which has assumed responsibility for the medical needs of the Indian population." Collier and the American Indian Defense Association, an organization dedicated to the protection of Indian rights, also supported the transfer, eying it as a means of improving care. Haven Emerson continued to label the Indian medical service "the most disgraceful apology for scientific or humane medical care" in the nation.[5]

The House Committee on Indian Affairs considered the matter and, in January of 1921, concluded the Indian health program did "exactly the same activities" as the Public Health Service, except it was nowhere "as efficient as [it] would be if transferred to the Public Health Service." Not only would the transfer improve the delivery of health care, the committee concluded, but it would also save the government money and provide a more "competent authority" to direct the health services for Indians. Homer Snyder (D-NY), chairman of the House Committee on Indian Affairs, saw practical reasons to integrate the two medical programs. Foremost among these was economy. That it would hasten assimilation and reduce the need for Indian-only appropriations was a strong underlying rationale. While the Committee favorably reported on the transfer bill, the House as a whole took no action and the effort died.[6]

Congressional Reform of the Indian Service

Encouraged by the chorus of critics (and the unfolding scandals echoing through the Interior Department), Congress opened hearings to examine the conduct of the Indian Service and to consider ways of further economizing the department. Melville Kelly (R-PN) chastised the Indian Service for "riding on the backs of the Indian." James A. Frear (R-WI), serving on the Committee on Indian Affairs, introduced a resolution condemning the Indian Service for neglecting "the health of the Indian until diseased conditions shocking beyond description have developed and now menace the white population of several States, while destroying the Indians." The Indian Service pilfered trust funds belonging to the Navajo, Yuma and Pueblo tribes for alleged frivolous or scandalous projects that benefited non-Indians, Frear pointed out, when it could have used this money to advance the health care of these tribes.[7]

When physicians Allen F. Gillihan and Alma B. Schafer were appointed by California Governor William D. Stephens to investigate Indian health conditions in that state, they were astonished by the "ill treatment" they found. California Indians had been reduced from 100,000 to fewer than 17,000 in the years since statehood (1850). Most were "living a hand to mouth existence" in homes not fit to be lived in and upon land that was of little value and lacking water. There was a "great deal of sickness" among the Indians, the physicians concluded, for which they received "absolutely no care." No wonder, Frear noted, the Indians were in a "hopeless, un-American and unambitious position," with the Indian Service exercising "unlimited control" over them. C.A. Harper, health officer for the State of Wisconsin, expressed similar concerns, noting, "reservations are filled with the most prevalent contagious and infectious diseases." The most important responsibility of the Indian Service, Frear argued, related "to the lives and health of the Indians." Property could be lost (and it was); civil liberties could be abused (and they were); constitutional protections could be denied (and they were), but "without health all the rest is of little value."[8]

Congress was dissatisfied with the Indian Service and how it operated. To increase Congressional oversight over the Indian Service, Snyder proposed establishing a statutory basis for Indian Service appropriations rather than funding the department through ad hoc spending bills. Since the establishment of the Indian Service, Congress had periodically appropriated funds for the "relief of distress among the Indians" but did so without a statutory basis. Snyder, concerned over the potential of piece-meal appropriations getting out of hand, proposed limiting funding to a statutorily defined list of nine expenditures.

The New York Democrat, who chaired the authorizing committee of House, opposed two appropriation activities that he believed violated his committee's jurisdiction. Foremost on his list was that Indian appropriations were subject to the points of order rule, which allowed members of Congress to make or challenge appropriations. If no one challenged a point of order then the appropriation was made—bypassing the authorizing committee. The appropriation of money without legislative authority, Snyder argued, was open to abuse and mischief if the authorizing committee were bypassed. Under the proposed bill, the power of the new appropriation committee would be limited while that of the authorizing committee would be strengthened.

The bill was largely a political play between two competing committees. Prior to 1921, the House Committee on Indian Affairs had both authorizing and appropriating authority for all Indian programs. When the House established the Committee on Appropriations, a jurisdictional tug-of-war over which committee would control Indian appropriations erupted. Congressman Charles D. Carter (D-OK) identified the fulcrum of the struggle when he noted, "The difficulty is that no general authorization has been made for many of the Indian Bureau agencies.

These appropriations," Carter added, "were carried along from year to year so long as the Indian Committee had jurisdiction of appropriations without much friction. But when all appropriations were concentrated in the Committee on Appropriations then the fun began." When the Committee on Indian Affairs lost its appropriation jurisdiction, they viewed it as "a clear invasion of committee jurisdiction."[9]

Not all members of Congress agreed that Snyder's bill to limit funding was advantageous. Several key members of the Committee opposed the bill as they viewed it as blanket legislation that would confer on the appropriations committee unlimited authority. Such a bill, Congressman Thomas Blanton (D-TX) argued, "authorizes, without limit or restriction, the five Congressmen on the subcommittee of the Committee on Appropriations to put into the Indian appropriation bill any and every kind of appropriation they desire to put in it. . . . Each and every one of those nine purposes [in the proposed bill] . . . are general in character and will take in the whole earth and the deep blue sea." With such authority, "the committee might decide that it was necessary to build a $10,000,000 Indian hospital in Oklahoma and likewise in each one of the numerous States harboring Indians."[10]

The bill not only appeared to grant unlimited authority to the appropriations committee, which Snyder hoped to prevent with the bill, but it also seemed to preempt the points of order rule appropriations. Points of orders were frequently used by members of Congress favoring assimilation of the Indians by challenging appropriations and indirectly halting the expansion of the Indian Service. Snyder believed the best way to control growth of the Indian Service was to limit appropriations to nine authorized activities. The Indian Service increased in size and scope each year, the Congressman opined, "until today there has grown around that little stump which started with the idea of civilizing the Indians more than 100 different bureau activities, including hospitals, schools, forestry, education, and a thousand and one different items." Every activity of the Indian Service already existed within the federal government. "There has never been a time when these various activities were added to the bureau under a substantive law, and thus make it impossible that appropriations should be made from year to year without being subject to points of order, as is the case in other departments, and under other bureau services."[11]

Congress approved the Snyder Act, as the bill became known, on November 2, 1921. Preexisting services were legitimized under one of nine broad categories. But instead of limiting activities, the law authorized broad legislative authority for an almost unlimited number of programs designed to benefit American Indians. The Indian Service was now empowered to "direct, supervise, and expend such moneys as Congress may from time to time appropriate, for the benefit, care, and assistance of the Indians throughout the United States for . . . relief of distress and conservation of health." The Indian Service had sweeping authority, as almost any activity could be included within one of the authorized categories. Furthermore, the law ambiguously defined the constituency to be served as simply "Indians throughout the United States."[12]

Emancipation of the Indians?

The programs administered by the Indian Service were affected by the ambivalence of Congress. In the wake of the Snyder Act, a renewed effort to emancipate the Indians from federal supervision and subject them to state and local law was initiated. Political and legal technicalities, however, impeded—and at the same time, went contrary to—this goal.

Emancipating American Indians from government restrictions caused much confusion. While proponents of the General Allotment Act assumed that the taking of land in severalty would dissolve the Indian's tribal nature and provide for his American citizenship with all its appurtenant rights and responsibilities, the Indian Service did not always follow such a course. In the end, two U.S. Supreme Court decisions helped define the position of the Indian Service. The issue that brought the citizenship question to the foreground was a deadly contributor to the ill health of many Indians: ardent spirits.

Alcohol had long been a factor in the declining health of American Indians. Colonial British policy recognized these problems and attempted to regulate the sale and manufacture of liquor. In the post Revolutionary War era, no federal regulations against ardent spirits existed, as Congress was content to let Indian superintendents curb any abuses that arose in Indian Country. Not until 1802, when the Trade and Intercourse Act became permanent, did Congress authorize the President to take the necessary steps to "prevent or restrain the vending or distribution of spirituous liquors" among the Indian tribes. Subsequent amendments strengthened the law, although loopholes allowed traffic in liquor to continue. In 1832, Congress completely prohibited all spirituous drinks in the Indian Country.[13]

Despite the Congressional ban on alcohol, it was impossible to prevent it from entering Indian Country. The 1867 Doolittle Report correlated the negative influences of liquor with the declining health of Indians. The situation remained largely unchanged until near the turn of the century, when Commissioner William Jones announced a ban on "illicit traffic in liquor." In 1897, Congress granted the commissioner authority to prohibit the sale of alcohol to any Indian who had received an allotment. Therein lay the controversy. As Indian lands were allotted in severalty, they were placed into federal trust for twenty-five years. Yet, American citizenship was immediately conferred upon the allottee. This posed a legal challenge as an individual was granted citizenship yet was legally incompetent to manage his own property. Since the Indian Service controlled the allottee's land, it exercised police power over him—including the right to prohibit the sale, manufacture or consumption of alcohol. When Congress gave Jones authority to regulate alcohol to any allottee—including citizen allottees—the commissioner initiated his campaign to eliminate alcohol, increasing the department's overall police power.[14]

The federal courts undermined the efforts of the commissioner of Indian affairs in a 1905 ruling known as *A Matter of Heff*. In 1904, Heff, a non-Indian, sold two quarts of beer to John Butler, a Kickapoo allottee from Kansas. Jones, acting on the premise Butler was "a ward of the government" subject to the department's liquor laws, pressed charges. The U.S. District Court for Kansas convicted Heff of unlawfully selling alcohol to an Indian. Upon conviction, Heff appealed to the U.S. Supreme Court on the basis that Butler, having been allotted land according to the General Allotment Act, was an American citizen not subject to Indian regulations and supervision. The high court agreed, stating the federal government was "under no constitutional obligation to continue the relationship of guardian and ward" and could "abandon the guardianship and leave the ward to assume and be subject to all privileges and burdens of one *sui juris*" at any time. Allotment meant citizenship, and citizenship implied subjection to state and local law. By court fiat, allottees were citizens no longer subject to the police power of the Indian Service.[15]

Congress, while professing the goal of emancipating the Indians, was taken back by its loss of authority over Indian allottees. The lawmakers' response was immediate, as they enacted into law the Burke Act. The new law explicitly postponed citizenship until the end of the twenty-five year trust period, thereby skirting the limitations on police powers that the court had established.[16] Armed with this new authority, Francis Leupp declared the suppression of all liquor traffic among the Indians had been "realized beyond all expectation." In 1915, Cato Sells instituted an essay contest in Indian schools, focusing on "What do I Know about Alcohol?" (primary grades) and "Alcohol and My Future" (secondary grades). The following year, he appealed to department employees to encourage and support Indians "in school and out of school, young and old" who pledged to refrain from alcohol.[17]

Sells moved to issue certificates of competency in record numbers after 1913. As more Indians were administratively declared competent and granted citizenship, the Supreme Court in *U.S. v. Nice* was again asked to review the question of the citizenship and the police power of the Indian Service. In 1914, an Indian allottee from the Rosebud Sioux (South Dakota) Reservation purchased whiskey and other intoxicating liquors in apparent violation of the liquor laws of the Indian Service. The question before the court was simple, yet complex. Was an allottee a citizen free of federal supervision? Or was he still subject to the police power of the Indian Service? In deciding the matter, the Supreme Court argued citizenship was compatible with both tribal existence and continued guardianship. Allotment of the Great Sioux Reservation, provided by a special act pertaining to the Sioux Nation in 1889, did not dissolve Sioux tribal relations. Therefore, the court held, neither tribal relations nor guardianship was affected by allotment. During the trust period Congress had the authority to regulate (i.e., prohibit) the sale of alcoholic drinks to Indian allottees. The Indian Service, as the agent of Congress, could enforce police authority without interfering with citizenship.[18]

While the *Nice* ruling was hailed as a victory by the fading assimilationist reformers, the Snyder Act was criticized by reformers. John Collier quickly became a leading voice of these new reformers actively working to protect Pueblo lands in New Mexico. Among the Indians, Collier found what he believed was absent in industrial America: a sense of community. Having visited the Crow Tribe in Montana, Collier spoke harshly of the Indian Service for seeking to undermine tribal nations by holding to an outdated "military policy which regarded the Indian as an outlaw and danger to society." Charles Burke's Assistant Commissioner, Edgar Meritt, refuted Collier's assertion, citing increased appropriations and changes in the Indian medical service. But while Meritt defended the Indian Service, Interior Secretary Hubert Work did not. In an article entitled "The Poverty of the Indian Service," Work admitted the Indian Service had failed to keep pace with "progress elsewhere along health, education, industrial and social lines." The difficulties facing the department, Work argued, resulted from years of financial neglect by Congress. Appropriations were inadequate to do the job, leading to stress and high turnover rates in the medical service. The whole department was infected. Teachers were hired who did not have proper qualifications, buildings were left in disrepair, good medical staff was difficult to find and even allotment was failing.[19]

To bring about reform, Work assembled a committee of 100 academics, social scientists and specialists in Indian affairs to make recommendations for improving the Indian Service. It served as an impetus for a number of substantive changes in the Indian Service. In a final report called "The Indian Problem," the committee made a clinical evaluation of the medical service, noting a "crying need for more hospitals for the general use of the Indians." The Indian medical service was "weak, where it ought to be as strong as it is in its school system," committee member Joseph E. Otis wrote in the final report. The tendency of the department to hire contract physicians was "the wrong kind of economy—it is saving dollars at the expense of Indian health and, perhaps, lives." The subordinate position of the director of the Indian medical service was a glaring concern. While there was a health program, it was within the education division with the medical director "little more than a traveling inspector." Buried in bureaucracy, the medical director spent most of his time in the field under the auspices of the education director, "who under the commissioner is the actual head of the Indian medical service." Indian health care appeared to be tied more closely to the management of Indian schools and the encouragement of agriculture and industrial pursuits among the Indians than to bettering their conditions. The Committee—which included Collier— recommended the medical service be reorganized as an independent division under the general supervision of the commissioner of Indian affairs. Agency physicians were to be independent of local, autonomous superintendents. If such changes were implemented, the Indian medical service might "function so much more effectively that Congress [could] be won over to the constant plea to increase salaries."[20]

Reorganization of Indian Service

A physician himself, Secretary Work wanted progress in the campaign to improve Indian health. Almost immediately, he reorganized the Indian Service by creating the Division of Indian Health and making the medical director directly accountable to the commissioner. Newberne now had direct access to Burke. Despite Newberne's opposition, Work added public health nurses to the Indian health program, with Elinor Gregg appointed as the first supervisor. When Newberne died in 1926, Work seized the opportunity and asked the Public Health Service to detail one of its medical officers to the Indian Service to serve as director of the Division of Indian Health. He then authorized the Public Health Service to supervise and direct the health services for American Indians, trusting the agency would elevate and improve the level and delivery of health services. In cooperation with the Public Health Service, the Division of Indian Health turned to state funding sources to supplement its medical shortages, something Gregg initiated when the South Dakota State Board of Health agreed to provide diagnostic clinics for the Sioux, an outreach that expanded the public health nursing program.[21]

At the center of the reorganization was an invitation extended to Public Health Service Commissioned Corps officers to assist the Indian medical service. When Surgeon General Hugh S. Cumming detailed Dr. Marshall C. Guthrie to serve as first Chief Medical Director of the Division of Indian Health, the Indian Service turned the first of a series of corners that culminated in the transfer of the division to the Public Health Service in 1955. Quiet and patient, Guthrie recognized the need to increase the salaries of professional staff. In short order, he secured approval to double physician salaries from $1,200 to $2,400 per year. Nursing salaries more than doubled from $800 to $1,800. Guthrie then worked towards a policy of promotions and paid leave, both of which attracted physicians to the beleaguered program.[22]

Guthrie gave the Indian Service its first genuine director capable of making substantive changes. He was given supervisory authority over all medical, dental, hospital and sanitarium activities and served as chief medical advisor to the commissioner of Indian affairs. Supervisory authority did not mean Guthrie had control over the appropriations made for health services. Since Congressional appropriations were for specific hospitals, rather than for hospital services at large, when emergencies arose—such as an epidemic or an overcrowded hospital—funds could not be transferred to alleviate the need unless special funds were available from other sources. Despite these handicaps, Guthrie was empowered to call on any of the six Public Health Service surgeons stationed in the United States—an action he frequently utilized.[23]

Work created four medical districts west of the Mississippi River to better serve Indian needs. A medical director oversaw each district, which comprised an Indian population of approximately 62,000. Two of the directors were furnished and funded by the Public Health Service, with the Indian Service covering all travel expenses. The Indian Service funded the other two directors. Each was given authority to investigate and advise local Indian agencies but they did not control any of the internal affairs of Indian schools, hospitals, sanitaria or agencies. While they were authorized to inspect facilities and report on the standardization of medical methods and facilities, they had no enforcement power. They coordinated medical and sanitary activities within their district, investigated controversies and advised physicians on matters affecting healthcare or public health matters. As importantly, they promoted relationships with state and local health officials.[24]

While providing physicians with a sense of integration and professionalism, the ability of the district medical directors to deliver effective leadership and make statistical analyses was limited by the large areas assigned to each (comprising between five and seven western states). When a scattered Indian population living on remote reservations miles from the nearest railroad or highway is considered, the challenges became apparent. With vast distances to cover, the time a director could spend at any one agency was necessarily limited, hindering his overall effectiveness.

The reorganization of the Division of Indian Health had additional effects, especially among special physicians whose duties focused on the challenges presented by trachoma and tuberculosis. Special physicians who treated trachoma before reorganization were fortunate if they were able to revisit their patients within a two-year period (if at all). The benefit of reorganization was the apportionment of Indian Country among twelve special physicians to deal with serious health matters. This allowed physicians to (theoretically) checkup on each of their patients at least once every ninety days. For regular physicians, reorganization had practical benefits, such as access to medical literature, textbooks and journals, all of which was previously denied due to lack of funds. Seventeen vacant physician positions in 1927, pointed to the continued long-standing difficulty of the Indian Service to attract and retain physicians.

Cosmetic changes in the health program did not and could not immediately eliminate the dissatisfaction most American Indians sustained and healthcare professionals experienced. Salaries lagged behind other government departments, attracting the less-qualified to the Indian Service. Poor housing—one agency physician lived with his wife in a ten by ten room within the hospital—and subordination to lay authorities in professional matters drove qualified physicians from the Indian Service. Work admitted that a salary scale that was more equitable with other governmental agencies was the only way to alleviate these conditions. Until Congress was willing to provide such funds, the Indian Service was unlikely to secure the better-trained physicians.[25]

Work and Guthrie together improved the nursing corps. Field matrons, who were directly supervised by agency superintendents and often emphasized their own interests in performing their duties, were phased out of the Indian Service and replaced by qualified nurses. The nursing corps was expanded to include four types of nurses. Graduate nurses were favored as they were graduates from accredited nursing schools and certified by the state. Traveling nurses, who may or may not have had special training, often accompanied special physicians and were skilled. Practical nurses had no professional training but were knowledgeable of health care. Public health nurses were highly trained and experienced in combating public health challenges in Indian Country, albeit not always in the most culturally sensitive manner. Several Indian schools, most notably Carlisle, trained Indian girls as nurses, although most Indian nurses ended up working in local hospitals rather than in Indian Country.[26]

None of the nursing grades was fully utilized due to continuing, chronic shortages of personnel. Among graduate nurses, less than half of the 105 positions were filled in 1927, meaning twenty-three temporary nurses were hired. An additional twenty-nine vacancies among practical nurses and six among the public health nurses existed in 1928. Table 8 displays the ratio of graduate nurses per unit of bed capacity in 1926.

Table 8

Graduate Nurse to Hospital Bed Ratio, 1926

Institution	Capacity	Bed Nurses	Graduate Ratio	Nurses Needed	Percent Deficient
Sanitarium Schools	510	6	1:85	51	88.2%
Sanitaria	261	4	1:65	26	84.6%
Insane Hospital	92	0	0	9	100.0%
School/Agency Hsp'l	934	21	1:44	93	77.4%
Agency Hospitals	68	4	1:17	7	42.9%
School Hospitals	670	11	1:60	67	83.6%
Total	2,535	46	1:55	255	81.6%

(Source: Institute for Government Research, 1928)

The chronic shortage of nurses contributed to long, demanding work schedules. Most Indian hospitals were small and had but one or two nurses on staff. Practical nurses were typically on duty twenty-four hours a day, seven days a week and only on rare occasions were they given time off. Since nurses were not well-established and lacked respect in some settings, it was not uncommon for them to be responsible for incidental work, such as cooking, cleaning and other household tasks—in addition to their nursing duties.

In her new role as supervisor of public health nursing, Gregg traveled throughout Indian Country examining health conditions and working to create a demand for public health nurses. Although she found the dedication of nurses and physicians commendable, Gregg observed the conditions under which nurses worked as intolerable. Long work hours, low pay and one nurse per hospital made life difficult. On her visit to the Navajo at Fort Defiance, Arizona, she noted, "a conglomeration of cases in the women's ward that shocked my nursing sensibilities. A delirious woman lay on a mattress on the floor because she was afraid of bedsteads. She had an open abscess over the spine, so wide and deep that the vertebrae was laid bare." In this same facility she found "a mother and baby, the mother with puerperal insanity, and in the far corner was a child with diphtheria. Two children with pneumonia following measles were there as well as a newly delivered mother and baby, a typhoid fever case, and a tubercular meningitis baby." Within four years, ten public health nurses were employed in the Division of Indian Health. Their introduction, however, did not occur without challenges, as Gregg discovered Newberne was not the only one who opposed trained nurses. Many physicians resisted them as well, believing nurses had little to offer that a doctor could not do. [27]

The introduction of public health nurses was perhaps the most significant evolution in the Indian Service to-date, as they made material contributions to the health and well-being of the Indians. That such nurses were detailed from the Public Health Service (and exempt from the civil service requirements) was a *coup d'etat* as many nurses applying to the Indian Service waited months to hear the results of their civil service exams and often took other positions before being informed of their test scores. In addition to physicians, agency superintendents tended to resist civil service nurses, preferring untrained local nurses since it was easier to remove them. Once a civil service nurse passed her six-month probation, she became a permanent employee and difficult to terminate. Due to their college training and experience, public health nurses handled medical situations untrained practical nurses or field matrons could not. Insufficient medical equipment and the opposition (and arrogance) of some agency physicians made life difficult for nurses. [28]

When Work assembled the Committee of One Hundred and charged it with making recommendations for dealing with the "Indian problem," it provided him with clear direction. The Committee acknowledged the U.S. Government had a unique responsibility to provide health care to American Indians but urged Work to "use whatever means [necessary] to quickly and effectively" meet the needs of the Indians, including collaboration with state boards of health. With the active support and cooperation of the Public Health Service, the Division of Indian Health initiated such cooperation. Guthrie ordered district medical directors to cooperate with state and local health authorities within their district and enlist state and local support in the campaign on disease. While the Indian Service sought aid from state and local governments in the past—principally in the field of education—most states dismissed the notion of assuming any responsibility for health services unless the Indians were tax-paying citizens.[29]

In 1925, eight states—Arizona, California, Minnesota, Montana, Nebraska, New Mexico, Oklahoma and Wisconsin—instructed their health officials to cooperate with the Indian Service to eliminate disease, particularly trachoma and tuberculosis, and prevent its spread. Several state boards assisted the department in surveying health conditions among the Indians. Minnesota, Nebraska and Wisconsin all maintained visiting and traveling nurses on the reservations within their borders. To fight trachoma, small traveling medical units were established in the Southwest where the disease was especially prevalent. More than 38,000 Indians were examined, with 4,285 requiring eye surgery and 2,863 receiving other treatment. An additional 13,858 examinations were provided in other parts of the country, with 718 Indians requiring surgery.

While improving health conditions, such activities were designed as much to divest the federal government of responsibility for Indians as they were to encourage the complete take over by the states of health care responsibility to all within their borders. To this end, Work and Burke faithfully advanced the Congressional desire for such assumption. "The State governments maintain similar agencies performing the same functions for their white population," Burke asserted, and "state boards of health . . . are in a position to assume these responsibilities for the Indians and perform them more promptly and sympathetically than the federal government." Having already moved most Indian students into public schools, the Indian Service attempted to do the same with health care.[30]

By the late 1920s, the Indian Service boasted of minor gains in the status of Indian health. The campaign against contagious and infectious diseases continued with some state involvement, and additional hospitals and sanitaria were constructed. Several hospitals in Montana were equipped with x-ray facilities (the first in Indian Country) and, in 1928, Burke was authorized to install such technology in other general and tubercular hospitals. The Classification Act of 1923, and its subsequent extension to field positions in 1924, reclassified positions in the civil service system and upgraded salaries for Indian Service employees, including physicians. While the increase in compensation was helpful, it did not create parity between Indian Service physicians and those employed by other government agencies. Burke, in trying to enforce economy and eliminate positions, actually increased both, with Indian health appropriations rising from $370,000 in 1923 to $700,000 by 1926.[31]

But while some people assumed any medical service in Indian Country was beneficial, the opposite too often was true. For those in the healthcare profession, it was no secret Indian health facilities were woefully inadequate. The critics were aware of these inadequacies and so were medical personnel. To the surprise of many, so were American Indians. "The Indians," Gregg explained, "did know that there was a difference between the care in the (Indian) hospital and the outside hospitals. . . . It was no trouble to persuade them to go to the hospital for surgery, provided it was not an Indian Service hospital." Even the Brotherhood of North American Indians memorialized Congress seeking to have an Indian advisory board to make recommendations to the agencies regarding healthcare. [32]

Renewed Criticism

If either Burke or Work were pleased with the accomplishments of the Division of Indian Health, they largely stood alone. Criticism continued to pour in from an assortment of organizations, including the American Indian Defense Association, prominent members of the American Medical Association and the Indians themselves. Haven Emerson was a leading faultfinder, condemning the "episodic and inadequate" care provided by the Division of Indian Health. Emerson was especially vocal in his opinion of Burke. The commissioner had a tendency to "create an impression that existing administrative initiative is sufficing to deal with a serious and tragic condition" when it was not, the academic Emerson wrote. Guthrie refuted the charge (and claims of an increasing death rate) but did acknowledge the challenges of Indian health were "enormous." To win the war on disease, the medical director conceded, required the "advice, cooperation and constructive criticism" of outside agencies. [33]

Burke resigned as Commissioner in 1929, partially due to poor health and partially because he was no longer effective in running the Indian Service. Two Quakers named Charles J. Rhoades and Henry Scattergood replaced him. While Scattergood focused on economic and property interests, Rhoades was responsible for education and healthcare. Before Burke resigned, Work responded to the criticism of the department in general (and Indian health in particular) by inviting the Institute for Government Research to conduct a thorough investigation of Indian affairs. The think tank completed its evaluation in 1928, led by Lewis Meriam and a staff of nine highly qualified specialists. Its 872-page report came to be known as the Meriam Report. "Taken as a whole," Meriam asserted, "practically every activity undertaken by the national government for the promotion of the health of Indians is below a reasonable standard of efficiency." [34]

The report was by no means revolutionary, as it was an amalgamation of existing research in the area of Indian health. But it was the concise and non-partisan nature of the report that made it impressive. Although the Meriam staff applauded the reorganization of the Indian Service, it found the department hampered at every turn by the "limitations of its present staff and equipment and by the lack of funds for development." The result was infant and early childhood mortality rates twice the national average and a tuberculosis death rate seven times the national average (with Indians in Arizona experiencing a death rate seventeen times higher). While an exact trachoma rate was unknown, it was believed to be very high. Despite more than twenty-five years of admonitions, Indian boarding schools were still overcrowded, regimented and routinized, adding to the high rates of disease. Such indifference on the part of boarding school officials to childhood diseases was most disturbing.[35]

In evaluating the health program, the Meriam staff found inadequate health facilities and equipment, unqualified and/or a shortage of health personnel, inadequate salaries and housing for health professionals, and a system of purchasing obsolete and outdated medical supplies and medicines from excess army and navy supplies. There was a pressing need for keeping accurate medical statistics as a method of combating the spread of disease and allowing a modern approach to fighting disease. An overall "lack of vision and real understanding" of what needed to be done precluded the establishment "of a real program of preventive medicine." The campaign against tuberculosis was ineffective and the approach to treating trachoma was perfunctory at best. Untrained instructors teaching health education and inadequate provisions for establishing working relations with state and local health organizations to attack disease and insanitary conditions supported Meriam's position of inefficiency.[36]

Had the report stopped there it would have been damning enough. Meriam found lack of attention to environmental matters that not only precluded a preventive health program but also made ineffective any program of basic health services. An extremely low standard of living and poor housing conditions were just two of many socio-economic factors influencing health care that were compounded by a misguided Indian Service. Improper (or complete lack of) sanitation facilities and an inadequate food supply compounded the situation. The Indian Service was so preoccupied with real estate issues that it ignored basic social and health concerns. "It seems," Meriam pronounced, "as if the government assumed that some magic in individual ownership of property [through allotment] would in itself prove an educational factor, but unfortunately this policy has for the most part operated in the opposite direction."[37]

The only hope of the Indians in their fight against disease was for the Indian Service to expand its medical services beyond the mere utilization of hospitals. To improve health conditions required environmental changes. The construction of sanitation facilities, provision of potable water and improved housing were essential. Medical care had to be improved. Additional public health clinics to identify incipient cases of tuberculosis and trachoma were needed. The two or three clinics then operating were inadequately equipped and too few to be of any substantive benefit. Furthermore:

> More and better-trained doctors and nurses are required. The plants of hospitals and sanitaria should be brought up at least to the recognized minimum standards for such institutions elsewhere. The practice of salvaging old buildings and converting them into hospitals should be discontinued. . . . Hospitals and sanitaria should be administered by

persons fitted by training and experience for that class of work. Patient labor should be utilized only when the physician certifies that it will not injure the patient and retard his cure. . . . The salaries and entrance qualifications for cooks in hospitals and sanitaria should be raised so that each institution has a good one, competent to prepare special diets and to serve well-prepared meals. For the care of bed patients the ratio of nurses to patients should be one to seven, and for the care of ambulant cases one to thirty.[38]

In short, the report focused on the need to create an effective public health program that could prevent disease rather than wait for it to happen. Public health nurses had to replace untrained nurses and matrons. Physicians trained as public health specialists were essential. State and local governments had to assume more responsibility for Indian health care, with the federal government subsidizing such services. Any transfer of responsibility, however, was to be cautiously implemented. "The sooner the States and counties can be brought to the position where they will render services and the Indians to the point where they will look to the government of the county in which they live, the better," Meriam opined. "[B]ut the national government must direct and guide the transition. It must not withdraw until the transition has been completely effected; otherwise the Indians will fall between two stools."[39]

Catalyst for Change

The Meriam Report was the catalyst in improving Indian health care, as many of the recommendations were implemented in subsequent years. Although Indian health conditions showed signs of improvement, they remained more than two generations behind the national averages. The real impact of the study would not be felt until the 1930s with the election of Franklin Roosevelt as President. In a twist of irony, a liberal Democratic administration and the Great Depression teemed up to provide beneficial changes to the Division of Indian Health. In an attempt to jump start the American economy and put people back to work, Roosevelt encouraged Congress to provide a series of federal work programs and direct subsidies to the states to employ physicians and nurses in the Indian health program. The Indian Service budget increased from $15 million to over $31 million. A special $800,000 appropriation was made to improve the diet and clothing of children in Indian schools.

Heeding the advice of Meriam, Interior Secretary Ray L. Wilbur reorganized the Indian Service into five divisions: health; education; agricultural extension; forestry; and irrigation. A technical or professional director with direct access to the commissioner's office supervised each division.[40] Real change, however, would have to wait until Roosevelt appointed John Collier as commissioner of Indian affairs in 1933. Collier set out to establish an Indian Service brain trust that brought science and government together and appointed James G. Townsend, Director of the Development of Industrial Hygiene at the Public Health Service, to head the Indian health program. As a critic of the department Collier had demanded change. As its new commissioner, he now set out to do it. [41]

Notes

1. Kenneth R. Philp, *John Collier's Crusade for Indian Reform: 1920-1954*, (Tucson: University of Arizona Press, 1977), 2-3.

2. "Indians of the United States: Hearings before the Committee on Indian Affairs on the Condition of Various Tribes of Indians," 66th Congress, 1st session (Washington, DC: GPO, 1919), 46-66.

3. "Indians of the United States: Hearings before the Committee on Indian Affairs on the Condition of Various Tribes of Indians," 46 and 53.

4. "Indians of the United States: Hearings before the Committee on Indian Affairs on the Condition of Various Tribes of Indians," 57. "Reorganizing the Indian Service," *House Report no. 1189*, 66th Congress, 3rd session, (Washington, DC: GPO, 1919), 3.

5. Hoffman, 493-494. Hoffman criticized the lack of pharmacists, inadequate dental care, no eye specialists and inadequate pay. The government had a treaty obligation—or at a minimum a "human obligation," to provide adequate health care. Ibid, 81 (September 8, 1923), 848-849. Emerson, "Morbidity of the American Indians," 229-231.

6. "Reorganizing the Indian Service: Report of the Committee on Indian Affairs," *House Report no. 1278*, 68th Congress, 1st Session, February 1, 1921 (Washington, DC: GPO, 1921). *House Report no. 1228*, January 25, 1921.

7. Interior Secretary Albert Fall was involved in a number of scandalous activities, including the Teapot Dome scandal in Wyoming. The Indian Service had its own problems, including Pueblo lands, timber scandals on the Klamath and other reservations, the construction of a bridge for the Navajo that benefited non-Indian tourists, and the general issue of competency. *Congressional Record*, 69th Congress, 1st session (67:4), reel 171, 5034, 5040.

8. *Congressional Record*, 5040-5041.

9. "Debate on the Snyder Act," *Congressional Record*, August 4, 1921, House of Representatives (Washington, DC: GPO, 1921), 4671-4672.

10. *Congressional Record*, 4668.

11. *Congressional Record*, 4683

12. 42 Stat. 208. The act called for the Indian Service to expend such moneys as Congress appropriated for the following purposes:
   - General support and civilization, including education.
   - For relief of distress and conservation of health.
   - For industrial assistance and advancement and general

administration of Indian property.

- For extension, improvement, operation and maintenance of existing Indian irrigation systems and for the development of water supplies.
- For the enlargement, extension, improvement and repair of the buildings and grounds or existing plants and projects.
- For the employment of inspectors, supervisors, superintendents, clerks, field matrons, farmers, physicians, Indian police, Indian judges and other employees.
- For the suppression of traffic in intoxicating liquor and deleterious drugs.
- For the purchase of horse-drawn and motor-propelled passenger carrying vehicles for official use.
- And for general and incidental expenses in connection with the administration of Indian affairs.

13. "An Act to regulate trade and intercourse with the Indian tribes, and to preserve peace on the frontiers," 2 Stat 139, section 21. "An Act to amend an act, entitled 'An act to regulate trade and intercourse with the Indian tribes and to preserve peace on the frontiers,' approved thirtieth of March, one thousand eight hundred and two," 3 Stat. 682. "An Act to provide for the appointment of a commissioner of Indian Affairs, and for other purposes," 4 Stat 564. Francis Paul Prucha, *American Indian Policy in the Formative Years: The Indian Trade and Intercourse Acts, 1790-1834* (Lincoln: University of Nebraska Press, 1962), 102-138.

14. *Senate Report no. 156*. Congressional legislation prohibiting the sale of liquor to allotted Indians was provided by the Act of January 30, 1897, 29 Stat. 506.

15. *A Matter of Heff*, 197 *U.S. Reports* 488-509. The court held that the General Allotment Act conveyed citizenship with the taking of an allotment, not at the end of the trust period and issuance of the fee patent. While the land was to remain in trust for twenty-five years, the allottee assumed all rights and responsibilities of citizenship immediately.

16. "An Act to amend section six of an Act approved February eighth, eighteen hundred and eighty-seven, entitled 'An Act to provide for the allotment of lands in severalty to Indians on the various reservations, and to extend the protection of the laws of the United States and the Territories over the Indians, and for other purposes'," 34 Stat. 182. The Burke Act made two classes of Indians. Those who accepted allotments before the passage of the Burke Act were citizens free of government restrictions although their land was still held in trust. Those accepting allotments after the passage of the Burke Act remained "wards of the government."

17. *Annual Report*, 1907, 26; 1915, 8-12; 1916, 60.

18. *U.S. v. Nice*, 241, *U.S. Reports* 591. In reality, the Indian Service exercised little authority over liquor prohibitions as the march for national prohibition gained strength and Indian reservations went dry.

19. Philp, 42-43, 81 *Annual Report of the Secretary of the Interior, 1927*, 12-20. Appropriations for the Indian Service increased $2,338,463 between 1923 and 1928 (from $10,316,221 to $12,654,684).

20. *House Document no. 149*, 35-37.

21. Gregg served as a nurse at Base Hospital 5 in France during World War One. When she returned from the war, she tried industrial nursing, training school nursing and hospital management, but "none of them really excited my enthusiasm." The American Red Cross, however, was engaged in a project to teach and establish public health nursing, "especially in rural areas." The Red Cross hired twenty nurses with experience overseas to teach the nation about public health nursing. Gregg was one of them. Through this, she discovered her calling in life. Gregg, 3-6, 25. Work hoped the Public Health Service would help the Indian Service overcome poor recruitment and retention of physicians and other medical personnel. The commissioning of Public Health Service medical officers to the Indian Service was not a completely foreign idea. On several occasions prior to 1926 physicians and nurses had been detailed to the Indian Service to assist in planning or carrying out special health activities. In 1921, for example, when a typhoid fever control campaign was implemented among the Navajo and, in 1924, when a trachoma campaign was undertaken in the Southwest, such details occurred. Raup, 12.

22. Guthrie served until being recalled by the Public Health Service on December 28, 1933. James G. Townsend replaced him. Gregg, 120.

23. Even after the reorganization, the Chief Medical Director had inadequate staff. The director's office personnel consisted of a stenographer, assistant clerk and a special physician, but no trained vital statistician to evaluate the medical reports coming in from the reservation agencies.

24. Lewis Meriam, *The Problem of Indian Administration*, (Baltimore: John Hopkins Press, 1928), 221. *Annual Report*, 1926, 1-2. The medical districts were in Albuquerque, Minneapolis, Seattle, and Oklahoma City. District medical directors assisted the "scattered and undirected reservation physicians" and enforced "the most modern and effective rules and regulations for the preservation and treatment of such diseases." "For Relief of Certain Indians: Letter from the Secretary of the Treasury," *Senate Document no. 148*, July 30, 1909, 61st Congress, 1st Session (Washington, DC: GPO, 1909).

25. Hubert Work, "Letter to the Editors," *Journal of the American Medical Association* (81, October 20, 1923), 1382. Marshall C. Guthrie, "Health of American Indians," *Journal of the American Medical Association* (88:15, April 9, 1927), 1198-1199.

26. Public health nurses were on loan from the Public Health Service and lacked authority, as they were not nurses of the Indian Service. Physicians could advise the nurses but felt "no responsibility for making (their) work a success." Gregg, 35. A.R. Allen, "Hospital Management and the Training of Indian Girls as Nurses," *The Red Man*, (4:2, October 1911), 55.

27. Gregg, 104.

28. Meriam, 248. Gregg, 124, 249.

29. *Annual Report*, 1927, 51. *House Document no. 149*, 2.

30. *Annual Report, 1925*, 20.

31. *Annual Report, 1928*, 55. "An Act to provide for the classification of civilian positions within the District of Columbia and in the field services," 42 Stat. 1488-1499, amended 43 Stat. 704-705. Laurence F. Schmeckebier, *The Office of Indian Affairs: Its History, Activities and Organization* (Baltimore: John Hopkins Press, 1927), 232.

32. Gregg, 38. "Memorial of the Brotherhood of North American Indians," *Senate*

Document no. 489, 62nd Congress, 2nd Session (Washington, DC: GPO, 1912), 7.

33. Haven Emerson, M.D., "Health of American Indians," *Journal of the American Medical Association* (88:13, February 5, 1927), 424. Emerson was responding to a January 8, 1927, issue of the Journal which painted a "misleading" perception that the Indian medical service was making significant progress in the war on disease and that the Indian birth rate was exceeding the death rate, signifying improvement. Emerson showed statistics indicating that the Indian death rate per thousand actually increased 48% between 1920 and 1924. According to Emerson, the birth rate exceeded the death rate by just 3 births per thousand in 1924. Guthrie refuted these claims by noting between 1920 and 1925 the death rate increased just 4.9%. Guthrie, "Health of American Indians," *Journal of the American Medical Association*, (88:15, April 9, 1927), 1198-1199. Guthrie specifically invited Emerson to visit his office and personally examine all information regarding its "medical problems, difficulties and plans for the future."

34. Lawrence Kelly, *The Navaho Indians and Federal Indian Policy* (Tucson: University of Arizona Press, 1968), 147-148. Meriam, 189.

35. Meriam, 10, 208-216, 244-274.

36. The fight against trachoma was largely fought by "providing separate towels in the boarding schools, displaying posters in Indian communities, and in a small amount of rather ineffective segregating of cases in schools."

37. Meriam, 7.

38. Meriam, 31, 312.

39. Meriam, 99-100.

40. *Indian Truth* (8, March 10, 1931), 1. Philp, 96.

41. LaFarge, vii-x.

CHAPTER FOUR

The Collier Years

Before 1930, the evaluation of the Division of Indian Health was that it was incapable of providing appropriate services to American Indians. That the Indian Service failed to fulfill the nation's humanitarian obligations was evident to all, including the Indians. Frederick Hoffman, another persistent and chronic critic, charged the Indian Service with outright neglect. "Thousands (of Indians) die for want of proper attention," Hoffman protested, "and thousands of others suffer dreadfully the consequences of apathy and neglect." Even the conservative Board of Indian Commissioners concluded "only those imbued with the missionary spirit" had any hope of surviving the difficulties they would encounter working in Indian Country. Hoffman was particularly cavalier in his view of federal policy towards the Navajo, who experienced an exorbitant death rate due to the near absence of health services.[1]

Despite pleas for improvement, the Division of Indian Health remained focused on the relief of the sick rather than on the prevention of disease. This was a result of cultural barriers and challenges that existed in delivering (and receiving) services and also a product of poor foresight and planning on the part of Congress and the Indian Service. The 1930s, however, witnessed a transformation of these bleak conditions into the first substantive changes in the Indian health program. Experienced physicians and nurses, once unwilling to work in Indian Country, were now eager to and used government work programs to conduct scores of health surveys among American Indians. For the first time, the Indian Service gained an accurate picture of specific health needs.

The overall budget of the Indian Service more than doubled during the first four years of the depression, with the health budget increasing three-fold by 1930. When Wilbur reorganized the Indian Service into five divisions in 1931, he provided the health program with direct supervision by a medical expert and granted the program line access to the commissioner of Indian affairs. A seventh district medical director was added, incorporating Alaska Natives, and state involvement in providing health services to Indians—subsidized by the federal government—increased.

In a macrocosm, the success of the Division of Indian Health was directly related to the level of staffing and funding. The availability of professional staff failed to match the demand for such services, making minimal medical attention virtually impossible to achieve. The funds needed to staff health facilities were never sufficient due to the parsimony of Congress. Chief Medical Director James G. Townsend, who replaced Guthrie in 1933, summed up these realities in an address to district medical directors, who were expected to "devote special attention to the working out . . . of improved medical and hospital procedures without increases of existing facilities or enlargement of personnel."[2] When cultural insensitivities and prohibitions to medical treatment were added to the mix, the challenges facing the program became apparent. Table 9 illustrates the growth of Indian health appropriations during the 1930s.

Table 9

Indian Health Appropriations: Select Years, 1928-1940*

Year	Appropriation
1928	$948,000
1930	3,062,100
1932	4,050,000
1935	2,981,040
1937	4,062,300
1940	5,088,170

* Excludes other federal depression era funds.

(Source: Department of Health, Education and Welfare, 1959)

A New Approach

The appointment of John Collier as Commissioner of Indian Affairs in April of 1933 ushered in a new era of Indian health care. Collier encouraged Congress to continue the reforms of the twenties by extending its investigation of the conditions of the Indians in the United States.[3] He established an Indian Service brain trust to bring science and government together to find solutions to the challenges of poor health in Indian Country. To modernize health services, Collier successfully sought the detail of James G. Townsend to lead the Division of Indian Health. He then closed six boarding schools in July of 1933 and, using Public Works Administration (PWA) funds totaling $3,613,000, constructed over 100 day schools, which he envisioned as centers of Indian administration and community activities. Using $1,735,000 from the PWA, Collier constructed eleven Indian hospitals and renovated ten more. He secured a $500,000 appropriation for medical services, which he used to hire part-time physicians, dentists and nurses. New tuberculosis sanitaria were opened in Albuquerque and Toadlena, New Mexico. Using depression era relief programs, Collier secured funds from the Resettlement Administration to provide 900 Indian families with new homes. While delighted with this progress, Charles Young, Supervisor of Indian Rehabilitation, was cognizant that most reservation Indians still lived in tents or shacks and nearly three-fourths of Indian families needed new or improved housing.[4]

One glaring embarrassment Collier sought to shut down for its notorious abuse of patients was the Hiawatha Insane Asylum, located in Canton, South Dakota. Opened in 1903, the institution had a capacity of 100 patients but was poorly managed and operated with obsolete equipment and limited staff. In the twenties, the institution was a special target of criticism, including Collier's. The asylum was "so outrageously cruel and injurious that we would deserve to be blown out of the water if we continued it," Collier informed Interior Secretary Harold Ickes in 1933. But closing the institution was not without contention, as Charles Lowndes, the most recent appointee to the Board of Indian Commissioners, blamed Congress for the negligent conditions at Hiawatha since it refused to appropriate the funds necessary to operate the institution. He did not, however, dispute intolerable conditions. Fellow board member Flora Warren Seymour traveled to Canton and found little wrong with the facility. Citizens of Canton, fearing the loss of revenue generated by the institution, and even some Indians who opposed the transfer of their relatives to St. Elizabeth's Hospital in Washington, D.C., opposed the closure. Nonetheless, Collier closed it and fired its director, Dr. Harry Hummer, because of "acts of needless cruelty." Among the complaints was the chaining of patients to their beds and locking them in unsupervised rooms. In so doing, Collier sent a strong message across Indian Country. "Misfeasance and malfeasance of extreme character" warranted the closing of Indian health facilities. The great need for services did not justify medical malfeasance.[5]

Expanding Services to Alaska Natives

In the midst of the depression the Indian Service assumed responsibility for the care of Alaska Natives, among whom the Federal Bureau of Education had haphazardly provided medical services. When the Bureau transferred the Alaska Native Service to the Indian Office in 1931, it relinquished all responsibility for health care in a territory where vast distances and extreme isolation made the use of health facilities difficult—if not impossible—to attain. Among Native villages where medical services were available, the commitment of time and energy to secure them was often prohibitive. Nurses made two extended trips to the villages each year, "one by dog sled in the winter and one by gas boat in the summer."[6]

The Indian Service assumed fiduciary responsibility for Alaska Natives with the passage of the Indian Citizenship Act of 1924. This act declared all non-citizen American Indians within the United States to be American citizens. In 1927, the Alaska Territorial court ruled that the Tlingit Indians were "naturalized citizens" and were, therefore, Indians under federal supervision. The Interior Department subsequently issued a ruling that the Indians of Alaska were also "natives of Alaska" and the term American Indian was expanded to include Alaska Natives, such as Aleuts and Inuits.[7]

The history of health care among Alaska Natives—Inuit, Aleut and Indian—closely paralleled that of American Indians. Epidemics of disease and disruptions of family and community ties all contributed to ill-health. The introduction of infectious diseases from Russian explorers had the same effect as did colonization on American Indians. While under Russian administration, Alaska Natives received exiguous medical care—and then only if certain criteria were met. Medical attention was provided to any Native living near Russian settlements but only if Russian health was endangered. More importantly, medical care was given primarily to those whose hunting ability—and thus Russia's economic prosperity—was endangered by ill-health. In 1867, Russia sold Alaska to the United States and, according to Article III of the purchase treaty, the United States committed itself to providing Alaska Natives with the same care and protection as afforded American Indians in the rest of the nation.[8]

Under U.S. administration, the care afforded was episodic. The vastness of Alaska, with its scattered Native population, and the relatively little social intercourse between Alaska Natives and non-Indians diminished, but did not eliminate, the need for medical attention. Not until 1914 was the Alaska Native Service created, being established in the Bureau of Education under the auspices of Presbyterian minister Dr. Sheldon Jackson. Two years later, the first non-school hospital for Alaska Natives opened in Juneau. Additional services were provided by the Coast Guard, then known as the United States Revenue Cutter Service. As early as 1886, the *U.S.S. Bear*, nicknamed the "Bering Sea Patrol," plied the Alaskan coast several months each summer providing emergency medical services. By 1916, the Bureau of Education operated its own medical boat along the Yukon River.[9]

When the Alaska Native Service was placed under the Indian Service in 1931, 30,000 Alaska Natives became subject to the jurisdiction of the Division of Indian Health. To facilitate this change, the Public Health Service detailed Dr. Frank S. Fellows to the health program to serve as the first medical director for Alaska, which constituted a single district. At the time of the transfer, there were six full-time and five part-time physicians, one dentist, fifteen hospital nurses and twenty-three public health nurses and other sundry medical personnel; seven hospitals provided medical care. By 1938, twelve private hospitals brought under contract provided an assortment of services.[10]

There was a sense of urgency in protecting the health of Alaska Natives. In his 1934 annual report to Congress, Collier remarked that a modern health program was essential to the survival of Alaska Natives. Dr. Vance B. Murray conducted three surveys and found the death rate from tuberculosis among the Natives in southeastern Alaska at 1,302 per 100,000 population, while that among non-Indians was fifty-six per 100,000. With money raised by the National Tuberculosis Association, public health measures were inaugurated to combat the disease in 1935. Additional funding was secured through the grants-in-aid provision of the Social Security Act, with funding distributed to the Alaska Department of Health. The tuberculosis mortality rate among Alaska Natives remained ten times greater than the non-Indian rate when the Indian Service initiated Bacillus Calmette-Guerin (BCG) vaccinations, in 1937.[11]

As new Chief Medical Director for Alaska, Fellows worked to secure better health care. In 1934, he encouraged Collier to construct at least four tuberculosis hospitals. "No progress was made in securing new hospitals so badly needed," Fellows wrote Collier, "especially for the treatment of tuberculosis among the Indians and Eskimos. No further time should be lost in the construction of hospitals at Bethel and Ketchikan, in southeastern Alaska." Despite sympathy from Collier, who a year earlier lamented to Congress the limitations of the Indian Service due to inadequate appropriations, it was not until 1944 that Congress authorized the transfer of the old temporary Army hospital located in Sitka to the Division of Indian Health. When President Harry Truman approved of a plan to construct several additional hospitals in 1946, Alaska Natives finally received the necessary hospital care. The Indian Service later acquired an obsolete seventy-bed hospital from the Navy and built a 400-bed hospital in Anchorage, in 1955.[12]

Transportation was a challenge in Alaska. To overcome this obstacle, the Coast Guard provided medical and dental treatment to Alaska Natives living near the coast or along accessible river valleys. Beginning in 1947, the Alaska Department of Health provided general health services to Alaska Natives living in isolated areas by supplying medical and dental care via the use of marine units. Utilizing three boats, health teams visited communities once a year, remaining three to five days in each village along the southeastern peninsula, the Aleutian Islands and the Yukon River basin. Maritime services, however, were only viable during the summer months when rivers and other waterways were accessible by boat. [13]

Similar to the Bureau of Education, the Indian Service struggled to provide health services to Alaska Natives. At times, it could not provide services because of exiguous appropriations. It also had a difficult task attracting stable, career-minded and qualified medical personnel. But, as with American Indians in the lower forty-eight states, the Great Depression allowed the Interior Department and various Indian interest groups to conduct health studies among Alaska Natives, each of which reported serious health concerns. With limited funding, little was done to ameliorate the deplorable conditions in Alaska. [14]

A Shift in Indian Policy

Collier's goal as commissioner was legislation that would protect the governments, property and culture of the Indians. Collier was convinced Western civilization was destroying itself and threatening the survival of the rest of the world with its emphasis on individualism and materialism. Visiting the Pueblos of New Mexico, in the 1920s, Collier discovered a way of life he believed was superior to Western life because of its focus on harmony and communalism. Collier found his social zenith and embarked on a journey of federal recognition of the Indians' basic liberties, the conservation of their lands through communal enterprise and the extension of federal assistance and public health measures to their communities. [15]

To increase efforts in the war on disease, Collier encouraged state and local communities to be more proactive in providing health services. To protect what remained of Indian tribes and to enhance their communal way of life, the commissioner found two sponsors—Senator Burton Wheeler (D-MT) and Congressman Edgar Howard (D-NE)—to introduce a bill he drafted. The bill—called the Wheeler-Howard Act—was a proposal that repudiated federal policies of the previous half-century by terminating allotment of Indian land and restoring the integrity of tribal governments. Collier viewed the bill as the first step in rekindling the positive attributes of Indian life while at the same time empowering tribal governments.

The Indian Reorganization Act (as the Wheeler-Howard Act became popularly known) was the most important piece of legislation since the General Allotment Act of 1887. Foremost, the law was *dejure* recognition of tribal sovereignty, which had been undermined by forced acculturation and lack of federal recognition. Under the law, Indian tribes could organize a government of their own choosing. This provision, in conjunction with the 1975 Indian Self-Determination and Educational Assistance Act, as amended, has proven most significant in recent decades as tribes contract for, and assume control of, health care services. The law also set into motion a mechanism for tribes to assume greater responsibility for their own affairs, which did more for the success of public health measures in Indian Country than any other provision. Using this authority, a number of tribes, including the Rosebud Sioux, began community health education programs, with tribal members educating their own people regarding the causes and prevention of disease.[16] Among these successes, community health education programs developed culturally sensitive programs and acceptable disease prevention that worked to mitigate resentment and disinterest on the part of the Indians.

In 1941, the Rosebud Sioux Tribal Council authorized precautionary measures to be taken by the tribal community in dealing with infectious and contagious diseases. The council acted on the belief that by outlining rules for isolating the diseased and prescribing penalties for those who brought well children into the presence of those with contagious infections, they could protect their people from the spread of disease. Mike One Star, appointed by the tribal council as chairman of the Health Committee, explained that health measures were more effective if they were grown and developed as the "Indians themselves desired."[17]

To further a long-standing tribal goal of greater involvement over the affairs of their own people, the Indian Reorganization Act also established Indian preference for employment in the Indian Service. The Secretary of the Interior established standards for "Indians who may be appointed, without regard to civil-service laws," to any position in the Indian Service. Qualified Indians were to have preference to vacancies in such positions. The preference section also had a secondary and closely allied goal of helping American Indians enter the workforce, as many had been denied employment in the Indian Service.[18]

Wheeler, as co-sponsor of the bill, uncovered one motive for such denials during a 1932 Senate hearing in Arizona. Listening to testimony from Dr. Henry R. Wheeler of Phoenix Indian Hospital, the Senator was informed that Indians were not hired by the facility because they were not as good workers as non-Indians. When asked why he did not hire Indians, the doctor replied: "You could, but they cannot do it as well; the standard goes down." The Senator did not accept this premise. If the Indian Service could not "get Indians to sweep those floors as good as white people and cannot get cooks over there who have been taught home economics in this school [Phoenix Indian School]," the Senator lectured the doctor, "it is time we do away with the Indian boarding schools altogether, if these schools cannot go ahead and turn them out so that they are sufficiently educated to do the work in these various Indian institutions." The lack of Indian employees was a poor reflection on both the schools turning out such students and the Indian Service that refused to employ them. "It is about time we found out why," Wheeler threatened. "We are trying to get this thing in hand and if you are not going to help us in getting this thing worked out I am not going to vote for any more appropriations until the Indian Bureau officials themselves try to help the Indians instead of firing them and putting them out of the service."[19]

Congress was clearly unhappy with the state of Indian affairs, health care in particular. Some members of Congress—while still wishing to see the Indian Service abolished, were impressed by Collier's foresight and plan of action. Empowerment was seen as the first step of ending the guardian-ward relationship. Providing opportunities for Indians to succeed economically could only be beneficial. As important was the progress made in involving state and local governments in the delivery of health services to Indians. But more needed to be done. A companion law of the Indian Reorganization Act had a more immediate and significant impact in Indian Country.

The Johnson-O'Malley Act made a direct impact on the health of the Indians by expanding health services and establishing the first politically feasible mechanism for involving the states in providing health services to American Indians. The act became law in April of 1934 after more than eight years of debate over incorporating state and local support for Indian services via the use of federal contracts. In 1936, the law was amended to expand the number of parties with which the Interior Department could contract. The amended act granted the Secretary of the Interior the power to contract with "any State or Territory, or political subdivision thereof, or with any State university, college, or school, or with any appropriate State or private corporation, agency, or institution, for the education, medical attention, agricultural assistance, and social welfare, including relief of distress, of Indians in such State or Territory."[20]

Senator Hiram Johnson (R-CA) and Congressman Thomas O'Malley (D-WI) introduced the bill that became known as the Johnson-O'Malley Act. Through federal subsidies and contracts, the Interior Department was directed to "arrange for the handling of certain Indian problems with those states in which Indian tribal life is largely broken up and in which the Indians are to a considerable extent mixed with the general population." In states such as California, Wisconsin, Minnesota and Oregon, where it was assumed that assimilation was largely a *fait accompli*, Indian health matters were so intermixed with that of the rest of the state that it was difficult to separate the two. The maintenance of a federal and state health agency for Indians in these circumstances was "uneconomical and contrary to efficient administration." The bill allowed "State health agencies to take charge of Indian health, and for the Federal Government to bear the added expense." Thus, there was an element of concern for the welfare of the Indians who were scattered among the general population (and for whom the Indian Service was responsible but not providing service) and an element of self-interest, in that uncontrolled disease among the Indians could become a menace to non-Indians. By establishing a mechanism for state assumption, the Indian Service could economize and eliminate duplicative health and social services. Nonetheless, Congress emphasized the transfer of programs was permissible—not mandatory. Both Ickes and Collier were quick to clarify the bill was not predicated on state assumption of services for those tribes who were still largely tribal in nature, particularly in the Southwest. State assumption with federal support would only take effect among those tribes if the Indians sought such cooperation.[21]

After enactment of the law, the Indian Service discharged some of its responsibilities for Indians, mostly in the field of education but also in the area of health services. Because of the unique political relationship between Indian tribes and the federal and state governments, Indians traditionally looked to the federal government for health services. This relationship was predicated on treaty provisions and the government-to-government relationship. States, due to the political status of tribal nations, regarded Indian Country beyond their jurisdiction. Therein lay the uniqueness of the law. It authorized states to assume the responsibility of providing health services to the Indians with the federal government providing the financial incentive for doing so. In the process, American Indians would look to the states—rather than the federal government—for services, furthering the goal of federal divestiture of Indian-only services. [22]

State and local cooperation in providing health care was not new, having been initiated prior to passage of the Johnson-O'Malley Act. In 1926, for instance, the Swing-Johnson bill intended to grant California authority to assume responsibility for providing services to its Indian constituents. Congressional representatives introduced similar bills from Wisconsin and Montana, although none was enacted. Nonetheless, Wisconsin appropriated $8,000 for public health work among the Indians and several other states provided health care for Indians if hardship prevented them from acquiring services elsewhere. Some states provided services since they did not want neighboring non-Indians threatened by the unsanitary conditions that existed on many reservations.[23]

By the 1930s, additional states expressed interest in expanding hospital and sanitarium facilities to Indian patients. Minnesota desired to expand the state sanitarium at Ah-Gwah-Ching to admit Indian patients if federal dollars were provided. In 1934, it contracted with the Indian Service for sanitaria services and within a year 117 Indian patients were treated on a contractual basis after they transferred to the facility after fire destroyed the tuberculosis sanitarium on the Leech Lake (Chippewa) Reservation. Collier used Johnson-O'Malley to improve health services to two other tribes in 1934. A contract with the State of North Carolina provided services to the Eastern Cherokee, while a contract with the State of Florida made health services available to the Seminole tribe.[24]

The Minnesota experience was one of the more significant accomplishments of Johnson-O'Malley in that other states followed suit and opened sanitaria to tubercular Indians or provided other public health services. Ickes not only contracted with state and local governments for health care but he also opened a number of Indian Service facilities to state use when surrounding off-reservation communities could not afford to build and operate their own facilities. In an effort to foster cooperation between the Division of Indian Health and state health departments, President Roosevelt issued an executive order repealing the prohibition of federal employees holding state, territorial, county or municipal office by authorizing Indian Service physicians to accept appointments as deputy state health officers. In such capacities, they enforced state health laws and regulations in Indian Country, which otherwise were outside of state jurisdiction. In the process, Indian Service physicians became liaisons between state and federal health officials.[25]

In 1938, at Collier's request, Congress authorized the collection of fees from "well-to-do-Indians" who received medical attention at Indian health facilities. Operating with limited funds, Collier saw such authorization as expanding the efforts of the Division of Indian Health and at the same time transitioning the Indians into paying for services. It was important, Collier believed, that Indians "contribute something to the cost of that service." Despite legislative authorization, the actual collection of fees was left to the discretion of the physician in charge of the local health facility. The authorization of such collection suggested Congress not only wanted to contract Indian health services out to state and local governments but was also interested in finding ways to assess charges on those Indians who utilized government services and could afford to reimburse such costs.[26]

The expansion of facilities and the inclusion of services to Alaska Natives added to the core challenges facing the Division of Indian Health. Collier was painfully aware of these difficulties, admitting that the medical service was "quantitatively, very much insufficient." Testifying before the House Committee on Indian Affairs, Collier explained health care appropriations remained "tragically inadequate." To remedy the problem, he argued the Indian Service should either "surrender its connection" with the Public Health Service or Congress should turn "the whole health job" over to that agency. The former measure was not feasible, as Collier estimated it would cost the government an additional $1,000,000 in salaries. The latter was equally unrealistic in Collier's mind.[27]

The Nursing Corps

Despite limited general funds, public health nurses increased in number after 1928. The ten public health nurses, for example, increased to 110 by 1939, with the total number of nurses more than doubling from 401, in 1932, to 805, by 1950. Despite the increase, the Indian Service remained handicapped by an average annual turnover rate of 80%. In 1934, for example, seventy-one nurses left the agency, with just sixty-seven hired, for a net loss of four. This far surpassed the comparable annual rates of the Army (7%) and the Navy (11%). Even as late as 1944 there were 188 vacancies in the nursing corps. In Alaska it was especially difficult to recruit nurses for duty in remote areas and, once there, to keep them on the job long enough to understand the nature of the local concerns. In what was becoming glaringly apparent, medical staff was slow to recognize, appreciate and consider tribal cultural concerns. An imposed system of medical care could not be one-size-fits-all.[28]

Collier was aware of the high turnover rate, and year after year he lamented the burdens placed on nurses. One major factor in the disparity of annual turnover rates was that nurses in the Indian Service worked on average anywhere from fifty-eight to sixty-six hours per week, while other governmental nurses worked no more than fifty hours. A patient-to-nurse ratio that exceeded similar rates in other federal agencies compounded matters, as denoted in Table 10.[29]

Table 10

Patient Loads and Nurse Turnover Rates in Government Agencies, 1934

Agency	Hospitals	Nurses	Nurse-to-Bed Ratio	Turnover Rate	Hours Weekly
Army	28	670	1:15	7%	48
Navy	19	330	1:20	11%	40
Veterans	77	2,700	1:8	7%	42
PHS	26	463	1:11	20%	50
Indian	94	291	1:14	80%	58-66

(Source: Public Health Service Bulletin No. 223, 1936)

Long hours, overwork and physical breakdowns combined with heavy peripheral work, such as food preparation, purchasing supplies, typing records, giving anesthetics, supervising the cleaning of the hospitals, issuing drugs and delivering babies in the absence of the physicians, manifested themselves in high turnover rates and made it difficult to maintain and operate an efficient nursing program. Given these factors, Collier opined that the nursing program needed "superwomen." Although Congress funded forty-five additional nurses in 1934, the nursing corps saw no reduction in work, even though Indian Service nurses were better compensated than other government nurses. For the first time, the Indian Service recognized that an effective health program required more than additional funding. Townsend gave voice to such thoughts in 1936 when he argued salary alone would not end the high turnover rates in the Indian Service. "After making allowance for differences in occupancy rates of hospital beds between the several Government services," the director declared, "it still appears that the nurses of the Indian Service have an unusually heavy-duty schedule. The heavy-duty schedule coupled with isolation and lack of professional opportunities appears, as may be judged from the annual labor turnover, to offset the favorable position of the Indian nurse from the standpoint of compensation."[30]

To remedy the situation, Townsend requested additional clerical staff so that nurses could focus their time on their professional duties. This required improving the administrative relationship of the supervisory and field nurses. Field nurses worked directly under the agency superintendent rather than the physician in charge or the nursing supervisor. While amendable if more attention were placed on supervising the nursing staff, administrative changes at the agency level remained difficult and slow. The challenge was nowhere more apparent than in the office of the nursing supervisor. Elinor Gregg, then in that position, was stationed in Washington, D.C., and completely immersed with matters of administration on the national level. Four assistants provided support but had too many obligations of their own to provide adequate support to field nurses. Already spending nearly half of their time engaged in administrative work in Washington, Gregg's assistants had little time for field supervision. "Quite obviously," Townsend concluded, "it is impossible for them to cover the stations of the service and render the type of consultation service that would be most beneficial." Despite adequate salaries, the Indian Service needed clerical staff to allow nurses to do the duties for which they were trained, something Townsend encouraged Congress to do when he requested the Indian Service implement a program of field training for nurses.[31]

Congress agreed with Townsend and, in an effort to bolster public health nursing (the number of positions was determined by Congress and dependent on available funding), the Indian Office, in 1939, established a new civil service position called the junior public health nurse. These nurses were not required to have nursing experience but would, instead, be assigned to an experience center for six months, working under the close supervision of a trained nurse. At the end of their probationary period they were assigned to fill vacancies throughout the health program, assisting professional nurses in hospitals, clinics and schools with administrative duties. In an effort to lessen the authority of the superintendent, these nurses reported directly to the trained nurses supervising them. While a novel approach, junior nurses never enjoyed a major role in the health program, although they did exemplify the desperate state of the Indian Service in trying to mitigate cultural and fiscal challenges in the nursing field.

Another initiative was the training of young Indian women to assist nurses. While not a novel approach—Carlisle Indian School had been training young Indian women as nurses since the turn of the century—the Indian Service established two five-week health institutes at Santa Fe Indian School in the summers of 1934 and 1935. Operated under the direction of District Nursing

Supervisor Sally Lucas Jean, more than 310 Indian women were trained by the end of 1935. Since most of the women admitted to the program were of marriageable age, the courses consisted of practical health care "with the view of preparing them—as wives, mothers and neighbors—to promote health and to prevent disease." Emphasis was placed on understanding the nature of bacteria, maintaining patient records, preparing food budgets and other ancillary skills. At the end of the second year, fifteen young women were employed as health aides in community schools on the Navajo Reservation. The program was so successful that it was expanded in 1935 with the creation of the Kiowa School of Practical Nursing in Lawton, Oklahoma. [32]

The Kiowa training school marked the first organized effort on the part of the Indian Service to train Indian women as nurses or nursing aides in Indian Country (the Carlisle experience was predicated on providing employment outside of Indian Country and demonstrating the successful integration of Indian students into the national polity, not training Indian women to work in their communities). Other efforts, such as the Santa Fe institutes, provided training in basic health care but more as a method of educating young women for their future roles as mothers and wives than as a matter of training practicing nursing aides. With the creation of the Kiowa School of Practical Nursing, the focus shifted and the program expanded from five weeks to nine months. The original objective was to train twenty Indian nursing aides each year, although by 1942 the school was producing twice that number to meet the emergency conditions created by World War Two. The curriculum included practical nursing, psychology, history of nursing, ethics, personal hygiene, anatomy, drugs and solutions, diet and disease, and communicable diseases. Graduates were placed in Indian Service hospitals to gain para-professional experience. In 1951, the program was expanded to a twelve-month course. Individual hospitals then trained the nurses to serve the specific need within their facility. [33]

In 1952, the Indian Service opened a second school of practical nursing at Mt. Edgecumbe Medical Center in Sitka, Alaska. Three years later, the Kiowa school was transferred to Albuquerque, New Mexico, where additional clinical facilities were available for student experience, including the Albuquerque Indian Sanitarium, the Santa Fe Indian Hospital, the Public Health Nursing Clinic and the Navajo Medical Center. A number of graduating Indian nurses were sent to Wendover, Kentucky, where they received additional training working at a rural health clinic. [34]

In addition to the school of practical nursing, the Indian Service provided educational loans for Indian students to attend nursing schools and become certified professional graduate nurses. The policy of the Indian Service was to provide "training in white hospitals by arranging for nursing scholarships, by selecting suitable high school graduates as trainees who have ability and interest." The graduate nursing school program typically accepted all Indian

Service-trained nursing aides as candidates for scholarships and, upon graduation, such nurses were virtually assured of employment in the Division of Indian Health. Well-trained to work in Indian hospitals, their primary objective was to "educate their people in accepted health practices." While health care was still defined in Western terms, the admission of such nurses opened the door to more culturally sensitive health services.[35]

Collier saw the success of the Indian nursing program justifying the Indian Service operating its own school of nursing. Arranging with the National League of Nursing Education to survey Indian hospitals to determine such feasibility, Collier hoped such a school could be established at either the Fort Defiance (Navajo) or Kiowa hospital. Despite Collier's optimism, the National League of Nursing Education concluded it was not feasible to establish such an institution since none of the Indian hospitals had the facilities, equipment or staff for such an undertaking. The high cost of developing such a school was a prohibiting factor, especially when Congress believed it was more economical to send Indian women to non-Indian nursing schools than to establish one specifically for them. Regardless, ninety-two Indian graduate nurses and forty-four Indian nursing aids were trained and employed by the Division of Indian Health by 1940, marking the first significant numbers of Indian nurses working in the program.[36]

Public health nurses were still the most noteworthy in the Division of Indian Health. When first entering the program in the 1920s, it was common for public health nurses to find tubercular patients turned away due to a lack of quarantined rooms or to see bones set "by guesswork." Surgical procedures were undertaken without room lights and bed linens were changed but once every seventeen days. "The hospital situation looked hopeless," Gregg wrote in 1936. "The more I saw of the substantial Indians the more I understood the hopeless tangle that their logical minds found in the policies of the Government." When challenged if her nurses could get the Indians to understand the importance of public health measures, Gregg responded in the affirmative, but noted it would take "a good grade of skillful care" and a "good many nurses and lots of visiting in homes."[37]

Owing to the efforts of Gregg, public health nurses had a defined mission in Indian Country: they were to educate Indians and their families to protect their health and, where possible, ameliorate family and social conditions impacting health status. All public health and social programs for families and the community were to be correlated with the nurses. Above all, they were to educate Indian communities in developing adequate preventive health measures. To a large degree, the success of the nurses depended on the cooperation of Indian schools, where children were taught preventive measures at an early age.[38]

Despite the training of Indian nurses and an increasing number of public health nurses, the health program continued to experience a shortage and a high turnover rate of nurses. War-time exigencies were only part of the problem. "As the demand for nurses by the military services and by other agencies has increased, the maintenance of adequate nursing services for Indian Service hospitals has become increasingly acute," Commissioner Dillon Myer wrote in 1951. "While a considerable number of nurses has been lost to the military services, other equally important factors—such as remoteness of station, long hours of work, and lack of educational, social and recreational activities—played a major role in the loss of personnel in this critical area." And if the challenges were bad in the continental United States, they were "really shocking" in Alaska, where there was a complete lack of facilities, doctors, nurses and money. "There are places in Alaska," Gregg told Collier, "where the nurses are too tired to be considerate of the patients."[39]

The Indian Service Physician Corps

Although the nursing corps epitomized the retention and recruitment challenges of the Division of Indian Health, it was Indian Service physicians that served as the nucleus around which Collier attempted to build the program. Like the nursing corps, physicians—excepting the depression years when staffing was at a pre-World War Two high—operated at less than adequate levels. In 1944, for example, the physician vacancy rate exceeded 30%, with 100 vacancies out of 321 positions. One position on the Rosebud Sioux Reservation was vacant for six years before being filled. Even when a physician was found there was no guarantee that he was competent. The physician at the Ft. Belknap (Montana) Reservation was unable to perform surgery but he "could see the Indians who came in for aspirin and cod-liver oil." But times were changing. When J.R. McGibony was detailed to the Indian Service hospital at Turtle Mountain (North Dakota), Chippewa in 1931, he observed the agency paying high rates for contract physicians to perform surgery. When he suggested to the superintendent that it would be economical for the physician to handle such procedures, the superintendent balked for fear the physician was incapable of performing surgery. Only after McGibony demonstrated that he could perform surgical procedures and "that the patient lived" was the superintendent convinced that he was indeed capable.[40]

An additional challenge created by high turnover rates was that doctors rarely gained a firm understanding of the tribal community they served because they were not around long enough to do so. Too often doctors entered the medical service with apprehension, resigning when other opportunities arose (this was also true in the nursing corps). Some physicians were temperamentally not suited for the cultural, linguistic and geographic challenges they found in Indian Country, becoming more of a liability than an asset. One of the objectives of the Board of Indian Commissioners before it was abolished in 1933, was for the federal government to include a test for employees seeking work in the Indian Service to ensure they had the temperament and aptitude for the conditions in which they might find themselves. Having surgical abilities was increasingly important as many Indian Service doctors found themselves in remote locations unable to avail themselves of medical consultation. Moreover, physicians rarely stayed long enough to establish rapport with the Indian patients.[41]

Despite shortcomings, some Indian Service physicians were instrumental in improving the health care of the Indians. Special physicians, for example, were instrumental in discovering the sulfanilamide treatment for trachoma abatement, as well as expanding research in the control of other diseases, such as tuberculosis (see chapter five). In 1939, Dr. George F. Frazier, a Santee Sioux and the only American Indian physician in the Division of Indian Health (stationed at the Yankton Sioux Sub Agency), won the Indian Achievement Medal for outstanding service.[42]

Like nurses, physicians labored under heavy caseloads. In 1934, 143 full-time physicians rendered medical care for 200,000 American Indians and Alaska Natives, an average of 1,398 patients per physician. This patient load was nearly double the rate of 1:740 recommended by the Committee on the Costs of Medical Care (the national average was 1:787). Townsend argued the patient load for Indian Service physicians had to be less than the general population "since they are required to cover such enormous distances over roads which are often very difficult to travel." The heavy caseload was exacerbated by the fact that many Indians refused to enter hospitals due to cultural prohibitions, preferring home care. In hospitals, patients were left alone while at home family and friends surrounded them. Even as late as 1949, when there were eighty-three physicians for seventy hospitals, the physician load remained high, with physicians being on-call twenty-four hours a day, seven days a week and eleven months a year.[43]

Despite salary increases, physicians were still underpaid. While not a new observation, the average salary for full-time physicians in the Indian Service was less than their counterparts in private and other government practices. Of the 143 full-time physicians, only fourteen were paid more than $3,500. In comparison, the average net income of a private practice physician was $5,467. Repeating a familiar cry, Townsend argued the "low rate of pay and the professional disadvantages of the Indian Service" made it difficult to attract qualified applicants and retain the "desirable employees."[44]

Heeding a recommendation made by the Meriam staff, and thereby easing a common complaint among physicians, Congress did extend educational leave to Indian Service physicians to encourage their professional development. Physicians were granted up to thirty days annually or sixty days every two years for attendance at "educational gatherings, conventions, institutions, or training schools," but only if the interest of the Indian Service was advanced. Although the qualifying terms of professional development restricted its use, the Indian Service for the first time encouraged it for its physician corps.[45]

Part-time physicians endured many of the same disadvantages as did full-time physicians, although the former could supplement their income through private practice. Contract physicians, however, tended to be more of a liability in that many favored their non-Indian patients at the expense of the Indians. Most contract physicians, even if they provided the minimum standard of treatment, took little interest in Indian community life and seldom participated in other related aspects of the tribe, alienating themselves from the people they were expected to treat.[46]

Consequently, the Public Health Service continued to assist the Division of Indian Health by loaning commissioned corps officers as physicians, although not until after 1950 did they constitute a sizable portion of the Indian Service physician corps. In 1934, there were just nine Public Health Service medical officers in the program, with seven serving as medical directors and one each as a dentist and pharmacist. Ten additional physicians had been loaned to the Indian Service in 1931, but all were recalled shortly thereafter.[47]

Depression era work programs aided physicians in their understanding of disease in Indian Country. In conjunction with state and private health organizations, physicians undertook scores of health surveys and studies to ascertain the extent of disease among the Indians. This epidemiological data proved crucial to finding cures or new treatments for disease. In 1935, the Philadelphia-based Phipps Institute conducted a tuberculosis survey among the Tohono O'odham near Tucson, Arizona, finding 402 of 508 O'odham (79%) reacting positive to the tubercle bacillus. In cooperation with the Cattaraugus County (New York) Health Club, a survey on the Allegheny Reservation discovered 78% of the Seneca testing positive to the tubercle bacillus. Studies among the Oklahoma Cherokee indicated 80% in need of dental care, 36% with diseased tonsils and 75% reacting positive to the tubercle bacillus. Among the Florida Seminole, there was an absence of trachoma and a very low tuberculosis morbidity rate. Additional surveys conducted among the Shoshone, Blackfeet, Chippewa, Eastern Cherokee, New Mexico Pueblos, numerous tribes in Oklahoma and Alaska Natives shed new light on old challenges. Coupled with the research of several Indian Service special physicians, these surveys made important contributions in understanding the nature of trachoma and tuberculosis, the two most destructive scourges in Indian Country.[48]

New Efforts to Consolidate with the Public Health Service

To overcome the obstacles impacting Indian health care, Townsend advocated moving the Indian medical service into the Public Health Service as the only viable way to improve health care for American Indians and Alaska Natives. A professional career health organization for physicians and nurses would attract and retain more qualified personnel. In a 1936 letter to Collier, Townsend outlined his basic rationale for the transfer. As the relationship between the several states and the Division of Indian Health grew more amicable and as the allocation of federal funding (i.e., Johnson-O'Malley and Social Security) increased and provided the states and private sector the incentive to cooperate with the health program, now was the time to chart the future course of Indian health policy. There were three options to be considered. The Indian Service could continue its current relationship, with the Public Health Service exercising supervisory control over the Division of Indian Health. On the other hand, the Indian Service could terminate its relationship with the Public Health Service and operate independently. But to Townsend and other similarly minded medical professionals, there was a third, preferable option: merge the two agencies, with the Public Health Service given control over the operation of the Indian medical service.

Townsend did not advise the continuation of the then-existing structure of Public Health Service supervisory control. The most pressing reason was that detailing Public Health Service officials to the Indian Service and granting them supervisory authority over Indian health personnel degraded the morale of the Division of Indian Health. As long as the Public Health Service supervised the Indian Service health program, "deserving physicians" would be hindered in any advancement to supervisory positions. Furthermore, because Public Health Service medical officers frequently transferred out of Indian hospitals to meet the exigencies of Public Health Service hospitals, stability and an intimate understanding of Indian health needs was impossible. On the other hand, the Indian Service was unable to provide adequate staffing on its own. But as long as the Public Health Service administered oversight, Indian Service physicians could not expect to gain such training, leaving the agency in a perpetual state of dependency. This was unwise. To withdraw the support of the Public Health Service would imperil Indian health and foster another government organization that would parallel the Public Health Service. "This policy is not sound," Townsend opined, "and it is extremely doubtful whether the Indian Medical Service could ever in reality be a career service." If the relationship were severed, the Division of Indian Health would continue as a non-career organization unable to compete with the Public Health Service for personnel.[49]

The only option in Townsend's estimation was a complete integration and merger of the Division of Indian Health with the Public Health Service. While the former was lacking much, the latter was "an old established medical service of government, well equipped through tradition and appropriations for conducting adequate clinical service and a high standard of public health work and research." The Public Health Service could provide staff with a better chance of promotion and with salaries commensurate with their duties. But most importantly, Townsend promised better medical care for American Indians and Alaska Natives. Fewer services would be contracted out, as Indians utilized Public Health Service hospitals where service in Indian hospitals was not available.[50]

Townsend acknowledged there would be "differences and misunderstandings" in both agencies if a transfer were effected. That was inherent in any government consolidation. Nonetheless, he encouraged Collier to initiate the transfer as "expeditiously as possible." If Collier needed a precedent, one existed. The Indian Office had once been in the War Department, but in 1849 had transferred to the Interior Department. While Collier supported such a proposition in 1920, he did not sympathize with nor accept Towsend's viewpoint. The difference between then and now, Collier asserted, was that the Indian Service had authority to contract services with state agencies. By pooling resources with the states, comprehensive healthcare might be provided for both the Indian and non-Indian population, fulfilling a Congressional desire for both economy and integration.[51]

In a letter to Ickes, Collier opposed the transfer, recommending the Indian Service be granted authority to employ its own chief and medical directors—outside the administration of the Public Health Service. Ickes concurred with Collier and, in a letter to President Roosevelt, supported the position that Indian Service, rather than Public Health Service, medical officers administer the Indian medical service. Collier found complicit allies in Ickes and Roosevelt and managed to fend off any further action that might have moved the Indian health program to the Public Health Service.[52]

In February of 1941, Townsend was recalled by the Public Health Service and, in April, was replaced by J.R. McGibony, who had been detailed to the Indian Service in 1937 to serve as hospital administrator. With American involvement in World War Two imminent, the transfer issue became a secondary concern, not to be rekindled until 1947 when Congress again considered the propriety of such a move. By then both Collier and Ickes were out of office and Congress contemplated the termination of all federal services to Indians. The Congressional desire to terminate the Indian health program would not wane until the transfer into the Public Health Service was complete in 1955.[53]

The Indian Service maintained its monopoly over Indians, successfully warding off a second attempt to consolidate its health program with the Public Health Service. In the process, Collier made no secret of his determination to retain control over Indian affairs—including health care—arguing it was preferable to contract health services with the states via Johnson-O'Malley. The Indian Service viewed itself (incorrectly it turned out) as not only more capable of delivering health services to American Indians, but also as more in tune with Indian needs. When Collier resigned as commissioner in 1945, the stranglehold of the Indian Service was finally broken.

Pause for Reflection

When Collier left office he was pleased with the progress of the medical program. He was particularly satisfied that more Indians utilized medical facilities and that some cultural barriers were overcome. There was an increased appreciation on the part of Indian Service physicians toward their traditional Indian healer counterparts. "Not only are [physicians] discovering the values in the Indians' medicinal herbs, massages, sweat baths, cathartics and cauterizations," Collier told Ickes in 1941, "but they are sensing a strong psychotherapeutic value in the songs, prayers, and ceremonies of the Indians."[54]

Collier also looked back with pride knowing he left the Division of Indian Health in better condition than he found it twelve years earlier. Substantial hospital improvements had been made. By 1942, twelve Indian Service hospitals were in the top one-third of all hospitals in the United States, a rating attained only after hospitals employed physicians and surgeons from recognized schools of medicine, provided clinical laboratories, x-ray equipment and lab facilities, and had the capacity to maintain accurate patient records.[55]

But while Collier looked back and saw progress, critics continued to hound the Indian Service. Former Collier ally Haven Emerson frequently condemned Congress and the Indian Service for their feeble and inhumane approach to Indian health. "Medical Science has the answers, but the U.S. Congress withholds the dollars to curb diseases originally given to the Indians by the white man," Emerson argued. Fred Foard, who became Director of the Division of Indian Health in 1948, argued further improvement in Indian health was premised on disease being "attacked on a nation-wide basis rather than sporadically and as a means of meeting emergencies when they arrive." Yet, the latter remained the Indian Service's approach for most of the nation's 400,000 Indian citizens. Even Commissioner of Indian Affairs John Nichols recognized much needed to be done, informing Interior Secretary Julius Krug in 1949, that there appeared to be "no appreciable decrease in the death rate among Indians."[56]

Notes

1. Frederick L. Hoffman, "Health Conditions among the Indians," *Journal of the American Medical Association* (81:10, September 6, 1923), 848-849. The Navajo resided on a 15,000,000-acre reservation and, according to Hoffman, died of diseases that the Indian medical service could ascertain only through "a matter of guesswork." *Board of Indian Commissioner Annual Report*, 1932, 29.

2. *Annual Report*, 1933, 80.

3. The Senate began its investigation in 1928, before Collier became commissioner, and ended its 23,000 page *Survey of Conditions of the Indians in the United States* in 1942.

4. Lafarge, vii-x. Townsend was detailed as a district medical director to the Indian medical service for six months (January through June) in 1927, before being recalled to handle a communicable disease outbreak with the Mississippi River flood of 1927. When he returned to the Public Health Service, Marshall Guthrie was assigned to head the Indian health program. *Indians at Work* (8:7, March 1941), 22. Collier, *American Indian Life*, (April 1934), 14. Willard Beatty, "Uncle Sam Develops a New Kind of Rural School," *Elementary School Journal* (41, November 1940), 185-194. Gregg, 14, writes that the amount received from the PWA was $3.5 million and that it took just forty-five minutes to spend it. *Annual Report*, 1934, 93-94. The Indian hospital at Tahilina, Oklahoma, was built using a $947,900 allotment from the PWA. "Medical News," *Journal of the American Medical Association* (107:18, October 31, 1936). *Annual Report*, 1936, 174. William Endersbee, "Soil Conservation on Indian Lands," *Indians at Work* (May-June 1945), 18-20.

5. Philp, 129-131. The annual reports of the Board of Indian Commissioners frequently contained health summaries in their reports given to the commissioner and Congress. *New York Times*, October 17, 1933, 24. Collier, *American Indian Life* (April 1934), 15.

6. Gregg, 152. There were seven small hospitals along the Pacific Coast for Alaska Natives, each with a physician in charge. Supplies were delivered once a year.

7. *United States v. Lynch*, 7 *Alaska Reports* 568, (1927). "Status of Alaskan Natives," *Decisions of the Department of the Interior*, 53 I.D. 593-606, at 596, (1932) and 52 I.D. 597-601, (1929).

8. *Final Report to the American Indian Policy Review Commission, Report on Indian Health: Task Force Six* (Washington, DC: GPO, 1976), 222. "Convention for the Cession of the Russian Possessions in North America to the United States," 15 Stat. 539.

9. Thomas Parron, *Alaska's Health: A Survey* (The Graduate School of Public Health, University of Pittsburgh, 1954), IV-1 and IV-72.

10. *Annual Report*, 1932, 76.

11. *Annual Report*, 1934, 96. *Report on Indian Health: Task Force Six*, 140. "Medical News," *Journal of the American Medical Association* (104:8, February 23, 1935), 662. James G. Townsend, "Health Activities in Alaska," *Indians at Work* (4:4, October 1, 1936), 7-10.

12. *Annual Report*, 1935, 140. *Annual Report*, 1946, 361. The Aleut hospital at Unalaska was destroyed by a Japanese air attack in 1942, just weeks after patients were

transferred from the facility (and the Aleutian Islands) and moved to the mainland. "Aleut Hospital at Unalaska destroyed by Japanese Bombs," *Indians at Work* (10:1, July, August and September, 1942), 42. *Annual Report*, 1954, 235.

13. Gregg, 164. Gregg wrote in her memoirs, "Leave Kotzebue in September by boat to Noatuk, 20 hours in a small native power boat. By dog team two days in Kivalina, return to Kotzebue by Christmas, 3 days by dog team. In January fly 12 hours to Shungwak. In February 5 days by dog team to Selawik. March—1 day by dog team to Noorvik and return. April—by dog team—detour and return to Kotzebue 65 miles by dog team just before break-up. Fly to Selawik—45 minutes—after break-up. One trip up river to fish camp in May." Parron, IV-33.

14. Townsend, "Health Activities in Alaska."

15. John Collier, *From Every Zenith: A Memoir*, (Denver, Colorado: Swallow Publishing, 1963), 93. Collier, "The Red Atlantis," *Survey* (49, October 1922), 15-20 and 63.

16. Collier, "Health Program of Indian Service," *Indians at Work* (9:6, March-April, 1944), 32.

17. Local political districts elected their own committees. Tribal Ordinance 592 allowed a jail sentence of thirty days or a $60 fine for anyone convicted of "taking a child or children under the age of 18 years into any home where there is any person or persons suffering from tuberculosis or any other infectious disease." "The Rosebud Sioux Organize for Health," *Indians at Work*, (4:8, July-August 1944), 8-11.

18. In 1955, after the Indian Transfer Act moved the Division of Indian Health into the Public Health Services, this provision was applicable to the Indian Health Service.

19. "An Act to conserve and develop Indian lands and resources; to extend to Indians the right to form business and other organizations; to establish a credit system for Indians; to grant certain rights of home rule to Indians; to provide for vocational education for Indians; and for other purposes," 48 Stat. 984. *Survey of Conditions of the Indians in the United States*, part 17, 8123. The Indian preference clause inserted into the reorganization act was not foreign to the Indian Service, as the 1834 Indian trade and intercourse act had also provided for Indian preference.

20. "An Act authorizing the Secretary of the Interior to arrange with States or Territories for the Education, medical attention, relief of distress, and social welfare of Indians, and for other purposes," 48 Stat. 596. In 1926, California Senator Hiram Johnson introduced a bill (Swing-Johnson) to allow for the transfer of some responsibility for Indian education, health and welfare from the Indian Service to the state. Collier and the American Indian Defense Association supported this bill. The bill failed to be enacted due to the opposition of Congressman Louis C. Cramton (R-MI), who rejected the idea of state responsibility for Indians. "An Act to amend an Act entitled 'An Act authorizing the Secretary of the Interior to arrange with States or Territories for the education, medical attention, relief of distress, and social welfare of Indians, and for other purposes'," 49 Stat. 1458. The law applied to the Secretary of Health and Human Services after 1955.

21. *Senate Report no. 511*, 73rd Congress, 2nd session, (Washington, DC: GPO, 1934), 1-3. *Congressional Record* (67, March 4, 1926), reel 171, 5034 and 5041.

22. The impetus for state assumption was heightened with the passage of the 1924 Indian Citizenship Act, which entitled American Indians to access services provided by the states. Most states found it impractical or were unwilling to extend health services to the scattered Indian population without some type of federal subsidy. Johnson-O'Malley provided the subsidy states requested and the discharge of duties that Congress advocated. Minnesota, Wisconsin, Oregon and California pioneered state services for Indians.

23. *Senate Bill no. 3020* and *House Bill no. 8821*, 69th Congress, 1st session, 1926. Raup, 19.

24. *Annual Report*, 1935, 136. "Medical News," *Journal of the American Association* (106:2, January 11, 1936). An annex at Ah Gwah Ching provided for eighty-seven Chippewa patients who were originally at Onigum on the Leech Lake Reservation. *Annual Report*, 1934, 92.

25. *Annual Report*, 1940, 381. In 1929, Congress authorized the application of state sanitary and quarantine laws in Indian Country. 45 Stat. 1185.

26. "House Committee on Appropriations, Hearings on the Indian Appropriation Act of 1939," (Washington, DC: GPO, 1939), 7-8. Sally Lucas Jean, "Health Institute, *Indians at Work* (3:4, October 1, 1935), 6.

27. *Annual Report*, 1936, 174-175.

28. *Annual Report*, 1934, 94. Parron, V-18. "Health Program of Indian Service," 32.

29. For an account of the life of one public health nurse in New Mexico for the month of April, 1935, see "Drama in the Life of Indian Field Nurses," *Indians at Work* (2:22, July 1, 1935), 38-40.

30. *Annual Report*, 1937, 236. Joseph W. Mountin and J.G. Townsend, *Observations on Indian Health Problems and Facilities*, U.S. Treasury Department, Public Health Service, *Public Health Bulletin no. 223* (Washington, DC: GPO, 1936), 18. Indian Service salaries for public health nurses ranged from $2,000 to $2,500 per annum.

31. *Annual Report*, 1937, 236. *Observations on Indian Health Problems and Facilities*, 20-21.When Congress reduced the number of nursing assistants from four to two the problems of supervision became more apparent.

32. *Annual Report*, 1935, 130-131. "The Institute for Training Navajo Nurses-Aides," *Indians at Work* (1:21, June 15, 1934). There were forty-seven Pueblo girls, thirty Navajo, ten Pima, three Maricopa and Hopi, two Sioux, Papago and Washoe, and one Ute, Mohave, Apache, Cherokee and Bannock. Jean, 14-17.

33. Gregg, 147, writes that the salary offered to these graduates was $1,080 and they "were in demand."

34. The first two Indian women to complete this training were Virginia Miller (Chippewa) and Adaline Clark (Oklahoma Cherokee), both of whom graduated from the Pennsylvania Hospital in Philadelphia before being sent to Kentucky. Elinor D. Gregg, "Indian Nurses Receive Training in Rural Health Work in the Frontier Nursing Service," *Indians at Work* (2:15, March 15, 1935), 15-16.

35. *Annual Report*, 1935, 131, 138. Elinor D. Gregg, "Nursing Care for Indians–Yesterday and Today," *Indians at Work* (4:4, October 1, 1936), 13-16. Gregg noted that about 15% of the Indian Service nurses were actually Indian graduate nurses.

"There is always an opening for a competent Indian graduate of one-fourth degree of Indian blood before a white nurse is considered." Those less than one-fourth Indian blood had to take their chances through the civil service examinations.

36. Raup, 13.

37. "Nursing Care for Indians–Yesterday and Today," 13, 15.

38. Fanny T. Marcus, "Public Health Nursing," *Indians at Work* (2:16, April 1, 1935), 30-33.

39. *Annual Report*, 1951, 356. "Nursing Care for Indians–Yesterday and Today," 15.

40. "Health Program of Indian Service," 32. Approximately sixty Indian Service physicians entered the armed services. Attempts were made to fill the vacancies but it was "impossible to find as replacements individuals with even minimum physical and professional qualifications." The Indian Service also lost physicians to the "more lucrative" private practice. Gregg, 36, 117. "New Director Appointed for Indian Medical Service," *Indians at Work* (8:10, July 1941), 9.

41. *Board of Indian Commissioners Annual Report*, 1932, 29-31.

42. "George Frazier Wins Achievement Medal," *Indians at Work*, (8:4, December 1939). *Annual Report*, 1951, 381. Dr. Charles Eastman, also a Santee Sioux, won the first Indian Achievement Award. Eastman was the first Indian physician in the Indian Service, stationed at Pine Ridge at the time of the Wounded Knee Massacre in 1890. He left the department soon after and entered into private practice. Later he became a world-renown writer and lecturer. Carlos Montezuma, a Yavapai-Apache, was another well-known Indian physician who gained fame through advocating Indian causes rather than practicing medicine. Montezuma worked in the Indian Service as a physician at Fort Berthold (1889-1890), Western Shoshone (1890-1893), Colville (1893) and Carlisle (1893-1896). From 1896 until 1922 he maintained a private practice in Chicago. He died of tuberculosis on January 23, 1923. Peter Iverson, *Carlos Montezuma and the Changing World of American Indians*, (Albuquerque: University of New Mexico Press, 1982).

43. *Observations of Indian Health Problems and Facilities*, 15. Fred Foard, "The Health of the American Indians," *American Journal of Public Health* (39:11, November 1949), 1403-1406. Congress provided funds for 145 physicians; eighty-three were employed. Foard argued a minimum of 250 were necessary.

44. *Observations of Indian Health Problems and Facilities*, 15.

45. 45 Stat. 493.

46. *Observation of Indian Health Problems and Facilities*, 17. Raup, 12.

47. "An Act to provide for the coordination of the public health activities of the Government, and for other purposes," 71 stat. 150. The Parker Act granted the Public Health Service authority to detail ten or more commissioned corps officers to the Indian Service. 64 Stat. 826. The doctor-dentist draft law of 1950 allowed physicians and dentists to serve their military obligation in the Public Health Service rather than in the armed forces. When the Division of Indian Health was transferred to the Public Health Service in 1955, commissioned corps physicians in the Indian health program fell under the provisions of the law. *Annual Report of the Board of Indian Commissioners*, 1931, 7.

48. *Annual Report*, 1935, 136-137. *Observations on Indian Health Problems*

and Facilities, 40-41. Townsend argued that the Indian community offered the "most ideal setting for cooperative enterprises by the several professional groups interested in betterment of the Indian life."

49. "A Statement Relative to the Past, Present and Future Medical Facilities Provided the Indians in the United States and the Natives of Alaska by the United States Government," *United States Code and Administrative News* (Washington, DC: GPO, 1954), 2932-2933.

50. "A Statement Relative to the Past, Present and Future Medical Facilities Provided the Indians in the United States and the Natives of Alaska by the United States Government."

51. "Indian Conditions and Affairs: Hearings before the Subcommittee on General Bills of the Committee on Indian Affairs, House of Representatives," 74th Congress, 1st session, *House bill no. 7781*, (April 2, 1935), 743-746.

52. *House Report no. 870*, 83rd Congress, 1st session, in *United States Code and Administrative News* (Washington, DC: GPO, 1954), 2928.

53. *Indians at Work* (8:7, March 1941), 9. Townsend served as Director of Indian Health for eight years. For McGibony's career statistics see "New Director Appointed for Indian Medical Service," *Indians at Work* (8:10, June 1941), 9-10. McGibony graduated from the University of Georgia Medical School in 1927. "McGibony Named Director of Health of Indian Service," *Journal of the American Medical Association* (117:2, July 12, 1941), 974. With Collier's resignation in 1945 and Ickes' in 1946, the Indian Service lost its direction. Collier's successor, William Brophy, was absent on sick leave for much of his three-year tenure. Brophy's successor, John R. Nichols, served just one year before he, too, resigned. Consequently, between 1945 and 1950 control of the Indian Service passed to the Congress by default. In 1946, Congress began termination hearings.

54. *Annual Report*, 1941, 433-434.

55. "Indian Hospitals Rank Among Nation's Best," *Indians at Work* (9:6, February 1942), 13-14. The hospitals were Cheyenne-Arapaho, Claremore, Kiowa, Pawnee and Ponca, Talihina, William Hastings and Shawnee Sanitarium in Oklahoma; Albuquerque Hospital and Albuquerque Sanitarium in New Mexico; Fort Lapwai Sanitarium in Idaho; Sioux Sanitarium in Rapid City, South Dakota; and the Tacoma Hospital in Washington. The American Colleges of Surgeons approved the hospitals. Of 6,291 registered hospitals in the United States, roughly one-third or 2,261 were accredited. "Indian Service Hospitals Gradually Meeting Standards for Acceptance by the American College of Surgeons," *Indians at Work* (5:2, October 15, 1937), 11-12.

56. Haven Emerson, "Indian Health-Victim of Neglect," *The Survey* (87:5, May 1951), 219-221. Emerson argued that an appropriations increase of $12.60 per capita for each of the 400,000 Indians was needed to control diseases. Congress granted a $2.67 per capita increase. "The Health of the American Indians," 1403-1406. *Annual Report*, 1949, 356-358.

CHAPTER FIVE

Trachoma and Tuberculosis

In 1931, popular critic Robert Gessner wrote of a visit to a nineteen-year-old Indian man dying of tuberculosis. Lying on his cot, the Indian lamented his condition and that of so many American Indians. "White man pay some day," he told Gessner. "Soon every Indian be filled with germs—soon every white man comes crowding around him. Then the Indian use tomahawk of revenge—tomahawk of disease. Then, someday, when white man's body all sick with . . . T.B., trachoma—he might open his eye." Walter V. Woehlke, editor of *Sunset Magazine*, also hyperbolized and stereotyped the twin diseases of the Indians. "In twenty states west of the Mississippi the Indian today is probably killing and incapacitating merely by his presence and contact, more white people than his immediate ancestors did with arrow or bullet or tomahawk."[1]

The election of President Roosevelt bolstered the campaign against ill health in Indian Country with additional resources. The increased attention resulted from the concern of disease spreading beyond reservation borders and a desire to improve Indian health as a prelude to final assimilation. No more significant progress in this campaign was made than in the areas of trachoma and tuberculosis. Improved health services and important medical breakthroughs helped turn the tide in the fight against these two long-standing Indian nemeses. Notwithstanding such achievements, an increasingly conservative Congress closed a number of Indian hospitals in the 1940s, leading one Oklahoma Indian to write Congressman Carl Albert (D-OK) that if the hospitals were closed, Indians would refrain from using state facilities because of the humiliating discrimination they faced.[2]

The Dreaded Eye Disease

Outside of tuberculosis, there was no more menacing disease afflicting American Indians than the scourge of trachoma, the "dreaded eye disease." Carried through the air and nurtured by the sun, the viral disease was easily and quickly disseminated. It thrived in the intimate, crowded and unsanitary slum conditions prevalent in Indian Country after American Indians were sequestered on reservations. No longer free to move about or relocate their homes, many Indians succumbed to the debilitating, contagious disease that led to blindness.

Reports of trachoma entered the annual reports of the commissioner of Indian affairs in 1900, appearing annually every year well into the 1950s. In 1940, the disease was described as "a years-long (sic) smoldering torment. It drives you wild with pain, unable to stand even the light of a diamond room without tears. It makes you feel, for months, as if there were big cinders in both your eyes, cinders nobody can get out for you." So merciless was the disease that it turned "eyelids outward. It may torture you by turning them in. Its slow inflammation causes wild, ingrowing eyelashes that leave you no rest. And if not skillfully treated, the chances are one out of ten that, when the smarting inflammation has eased at last, then the night has fallen for you always."[3]

The incidence of trachoma was unknown prior to 1912, when the Public Health Service evaluated its prevalence in Indian Country. Of the 39,321 Indians examined, 23% were trachomatous, leading the Public Health Service to conclude trachoma was "exceedingly prevalent among the Indians." Between 1927 and 1931, another study evaluated 17,320 Indians, with 1,213 (7%) having the disease. But the rates were never constant. The Navajo Nation had an incidence rate exceeding 30% while the Seminole Nation in Florida and the Taholah Tribe from Neah Bay, Washington, were free of the disease. A 1935 study indicated trachoma was virtually non-existent among Wisconsin tribes, the Eastern Cherokee and the Minnesota Chippewa. Indians in Oklahoma showed an overall incidence rate of about 5%, while the incidence of trachoma among the Mission tribes of California was less than 4%. No region was immune. While Zuni Pueblo had an incidence rate of 1%, the rate at Laguna Pueblo approached 25%. And while the San Carlos and White Mountain Apache tribes in Arizona had an incidence rate of nearly 30%, the rate among the Jicarilla Apache in northern New Mexico was just 1%. The same was true in the Pacific Northwest, where tribes west of the Cascade Mountains had little or no trachoma, but those east of the mountains (Flathead, Crow and Blackfeet) had incidence rates of 20% or higher. In 1939, Dr. Harry S. Gradle, an Interior Department appointee to the Indian Service advisory committee on trachoma, estimated there were 33,800 cases of trachoma nationwide among non-Indians (population of 123,202,624) and approximately 24,000 cases among American Indians (population of 350,000).[4]

The propensity of trachoma, a chronic, contagious disease of the conjunctiva, to afflict American Indians far in excess of non-Indians was nothing short of phenomenal. Effective treatment of the disease proved unsuccessful until the late 1930s, when Dr. Fred Loe of the Indian medical service discovered a sulfanilamide treatment that appeared to cure the disease. After 1939, the incidence rate of trachoma declined from over 20% of American Indians to 7% by 1943. The disease was by no means eradicated, however, as in 1955 the Indian trachoma rate per 100,000 was 280, while the non-Indian rate was just 0.5.[5]

The Indian Service first targeted trachoma in 1909, when Francis Leupp requested expert advice from Surgeon General Walter Wyman. Wyman explained the disease, while not fatal, posed a grave danger to the public if not controlled. "The onset of the disease may be so severe as to compromise the vision from the outset," the surgeon general wrote. "There may be ulcerations of the cornea and perforation and evacuation of the contents of the eyeball. Corneal complications almost always appear in some stage of the disease, unless ameliorated by treatment." Even if these consequences were avoided, the disease "almost always results in cicatricial contraction of the lids, which results in entropion, or incurvature of the margin of the lids, bringing the eyelashes into contact with the eyeball, and keeping up a constant irritation which results in corneal opacity, causing blindness." Acknowledging that it was easier to prevent trachoma than to cure it, Wyman warned Leupp "no time should be lost or no effort spared to eradicate the condition."[6]

The first steps in the campaign against trachoma began in 1912, when the disease was one of three that Congress authorized the Public Health Service to investigate. Even with convincing evidence of its prevalence, little improvement was made in the campaign against the disease because of untrained personnel, lack of funding and an unclear understanding of treatment. In an effort to prevent the spread of disease among children, the Public Health Service recommended the Indian Service construct a trachoma school where all infected Indian children could be sent to protect the health of uninfected children and provide limited treatment for those infected. Despite knowledge that Indian schools were the source of disease, the Indian Service did not establish a trachoma school until 1927, when two schools for trachomatous children were established among the Navajo at Fort Defiance, Arizona, and Tohatchi, New Mexico.[7]

The Fox Technique

With the high incidence of disease, Indian Service physicians began medically and surgically treating trachomatous patients using an assortment of home remedies, none of which met with much success. In 1924, however, the Indian health program adopted a new procedure for treating trachoma developed by ophthalmologist Dr. L. Webster Fox of the University of Pennsylvania Medical School. Fox believed the cure for trachoma lie in a tarsectomy. Despite inconclusive evidence, Chief Medical Officer Robert E. Lee Newberne approved the procedure for use in Indian Country. The tarsectomy, a radical procedure that surgically removed the dense connective tissue that serves to stiffen the eyelid, was based on indecisive research conducted among the Blackfeet Tribe in Montana. Blackfeet children, having been surgically treated for trachoma while attending Carlisle Indian School in the 1910s, were reexamined in 1923 during the course of the first trachoma survey undertaken on the Blackfeet Reservation. From all appearances, those children who had undergone a tarsectomy were cured. The Board of Indian Commissioners hailed the process as an "unquestionable success" that warranted "the strong hope that in a comparatively few years our Indian people will be clear eyed." By shear faith, the Indian Service was convinced the disease would be eradicated within a few years. Almost immediately, Newberne hand selected a number of physicians to assist and learn from Fox the surgical procedure hailed as the cure for trachoma.[8]

The next step for Newberne was to extend the procedure to all Indian Service physicians. In June 1925, Commissioner Burke issued Circular no. 2122 ordering all surgeons "to perform the approved operation for the cure of trachoma." Several months later, Burke issued Circular no. 2147, ordering all physicians to learn the methods of treating trachoma and performing the operation "recommended by Dr. Fox and other eminent ophthalmologists." Every physician was to become a trachoma specialist. The Indian Service performed thousands of tarsectomies in a "whirlwind campaign" against the disease. Physicians not properly trained for such a procedure soon performed tarsectomies, regardless of whether the circumstances required it. Indian patients were informed the procedure created an immunity to the disease when, in fact, it did not. Follow-up treatment to insure success was rare, resulting in blindness for many Indian patients.[9]

The tarsectomy was not a cure for trachoma. In September of 1927, Guthrie ordered the suspension of the procedure, absent special permission from Washington. Discontinuing the operation, however, did not occur soon enough for Dr. Herbert Edwards of the Meriam staff, also discovered 49% of all tarsectomy patients at Fort Totten Indian School, in 1926, required additional treatment. "Because of the numerous defects in the medical service," Lewis Meriam wrote, "serious errors have been made in the treatment of Indians suffering from trachoma." Meriam decried the callousness of the Indian Service for ignoring the close relationship between trachoma and dietary deficiencies and for pinning "its faith on a serious, radical operation for cure without carefully watching results and checking the degree of success achieved." Malfeasance was sure to occur with an agency "so seriously understaffed that following up cases and checking results are neglected." The result was the procedure was "performed on Indians who did not need it, and, because of the difficulties in diagnosis of trachoma, upon some Indians who did not even have the disease."[10]

The Indian Service was severely chastised for its uncritical acceptance of the Fox technique. It was also reproved for failing to provide follow-up treatment to verify if the surgical procedure was, in fact, effective. Meriam suggested trachoma was a deficiency disease, rather than a contagion, and chastened the Indian Service (incorrectly as it turned out) for not treating it as such. The Indian Service immediately discontinued the procedure.[11]

With Collier's appointment of an Indian Service brain trust, the first break-through in the campaign against trachoma was attained. With large numbers of trachomatous children on the Fort Apache (Arizona) Reservation, Collier converted Theodore Roosevelt Boarding School into a trachoma school and research center, in 1934. He then struck an agreement with Columbia University to send a trachoma expert named Dr. Phillips Thygeson to Ft. Apache in a joint Indian Service and Columbia University venture. A team of trachoma specialists, including Dr. Polk Richards (medical director in charge of trachoma activities) and Dr. F. I. Proctor (consultant on trachoma), was assigned to the school to conduct research into the etiology and pathology of the disease. An intensive prevention and therapeutic program was implemented to treat trachomatous patients. Working with an experienced and well-trained staff, Thygeson made an important breakthrough, in 1937, when he discovered a filterable virus caused trachoma.[12]

In finding a viral connection, Thygeson went back to 1912 when French physician Charles Nicolle demonstrated a viral connection to trachoma. In the United States this discovery was obscured by the claims of Dr. Anna Williams, of the Rockefeller Institute, who argued the disease was caused by a bacillus granulosis (bacteria). It was under this assumption that the tarsectomy was approved. In 1935, Thygeson used microbe-proof filters to transfer the eye disease from Apache children to baboons. Fearing baboons might react differently than humans, Thygeson and his staff sought a human guinea pig to serve as an experimental participant. In Iowa City, Iowa, they found their man: Clarence Brown, who had already lost his left eye to cancer. Thygeson invited Brown to serve as their human trial but promised no cure should he become infected. He warned Brown that he could lose his remaining eye over painful months of treatment. When Brown consented, the medical staff set out to prove the viral origin of trachoma.[13]

Using airmailed "trachomatous poison" sent from Fort Apache to Iowa City, the physicians three times failed to infect Brown. Only after a visit to Arizona was Brown successfully infected with trachoma. Thygeson and his associates then proved Nicolle's viral theory. After two years of drawn out copper-sulfate treatment, Brown was cured of trachoma. In an address to the American Medical Association, in 1938, Thygeson opined trachoma was a viral disease and that "its epithelial cell inclusive consists of masses of virus embodied in a matrix consisting largely of glycogen."[14]

To better facilitate research, Interior Secretary Harold Ickes established a special trachoma advisory committee in the fall of 1937. The purpose of the committee was to find ways to better wage war against trachoma. Among the issues examined were minimum qualifications for special physicians, the proper role of nurses and teachers in treating trachoma and finding ways to better maintain records to track the disease. Within two years, the Division of Indian Health employed twelve special physicians and nineteen nurses working under the direction of Polk Richards, Medical Director in charge of trachoma activities.[15]

Discovery of Sulfanilamide Treatment

Working simultaneously, another team of specialists was led by twenty-year Indian Service veteran Dr. Fred Loe, a physician among the Rosebud Sioux. Loe witnessed all the alleged cures from "iodine to chaulmoogra oil" and observed that individuals treated with copper sulphate or silver nitrate apparently healed only to have their condition flare up again, worse than ever. He examined patients "no better and no worse" after treatment except "they very slowly went blind as nature healed the inflammation." Loe informed medical director Townsend that he had trachoma cases that resisted every type of treatment. Having heard of a new chemical magic called sulfanilamide, Loe in desperation thought, "Why not try it on trachoma?" Research indicated sulfanilamide killed bacteria and Loe sought to determine if it would do the same with a viral infection. Since sulfanilamide was a compound of sulfanilic acid and is an organic bacteria-inhibiting drug, Loe theorized it would prevent the growth of the virus causing trachoma. Townsend reminded him that there were side effects, including severe headaches, dizziness, vomiting and fever.[16]

With Townsend's blessing, Loe selected two patients (ages forty-seven and fifty-two) from Rosebud. One had been trachomatous since 1932 and the other from childhood. In August of 1937, the two patients were administered an oral prescription consisting of one-third of a grain of sulfanilamide with an equal amount of sodium bicarbonate for ten days. The dosage was then reduced to one-quarter of a grain for fourteen days. Within twenty-four hours both patients lost their aversion to light and the inflammation disappeared, with the tears no longer flowing. After five days of treatment, Loe noted significant improvement. "It was truly wonderful the way those eyes cleared up," the physician informed Townsend, "and they did so in about two weeks." Within a month, both patients were discharged and after six months neither had any recurrence of trachoma.[17]

Loe then treated an additional thirteen patients and found the new drug to be the "most wonderful treatment" for trachoma. An oral administration of sulfanilamide seemed to cure (or at least arrest) the disease. While Loe acknowledged these cases were too few to conclusively argue that sulfanilamide cured the disease, Trachoma Director Polk Richards visited Loe and agreed there was merit in further studies. Loe's discovery stimulated additional research at Fort Apache where experiments conducted on baboons verified that trachoma could be arrested using sulfanilamide.[18]

Although Loe's original research was conducted on just two patients, it was expanded to 140 Sioux patients—ninety-three of whom were boarding school children—in 1938, all of whom experienced either abatement or improvement in their condition. Within twenty-four hours there was a cessation of lacrimation and loss of photophobia, and within seventy-two hours there was improved eyesight. Five months later, just twelve of the patients showed any sign of trachoma. This larger study prompted Gradle to implement tests of his own on a group of twenty-five non-Indians from southern Illinois, where he concluded the use of sulfanilamide appeared to be a "new means of combating the more acute stages of trachoma."[19]

Continued research in 1939 led Collier to announce that experimentation with sulfanilamide "far exceeded the most optimistic expectations." He authorized additional studies to be conducted at eleven agencies across Indian Country. Included in this expanded study were 122 Navajo children from Arizona and New Mexico, among whom trachoma was especially prevalent. Of 1,023 Indians starting treatment (excluding those from Fort Apache), 961 completed it, with 413, or 43%, having the disease arrested within three weeks. An additional 481 or 50% showed improvement. Of this group, an additional 122 had the disease arrested with a second treatment.[20]

Loe, meanwhile, expanded his test group to 202 Rosebud Sioux and after eighteen months reexamined each member of the group. He found the disease arrested in 196 patients, with the remaining six showing signs of improvement. Another 162 patients were treated on the Winnebago (Nebraska) Reservation and, of the ninety-eight who were re-examined, eighty-seven were free of trachoma, eight showed improvement and three were unchanged. Among the Apache children at Theodore Roosevelt Boarding School, 167 were treated with sulfanilamide for three weeks, with 125 (75%) having the disease arrested. With an additional three weeks of therapy, the disease was arrested in the remaining forty-two students.[21]

When the final report on the effects of sulfanilamide was made public, Townsend reported 70% of the 1,300 patients treated showed a complete arrestment of the disease. By 1941, Collier boasted of a "spectacular reduction" in the incidence rate of trachoma. In fact, between 1938 and 1943, the trachoma incidence rate fell from 18.9% of the Indian population to 4%. As the rate fell, the Indian Service focused more time and energy on trachomatous adults and pre-school children, even opening a trachoma camp on the Warm Springs (Oregon) Reservation after the hospital was filled to capacity. Polk Richards administered the facility, which was staffed by trachoma specialists. So successful was the work that by the early 1940s, the Indian health program no longer viewed trachoma as a major concern, although it did retain two special physicians to instruct new appointees to the Indian Service in diagnosing and treating trachoma.[22]

Although the trachoma incidence rate declined, American involvement in World War Two cut short long-term advances in treatment and research. The pressures of fighting the war on two fronts compelled the United States to decrease funding for social programs—including the Indian Service—and convert it to wartime industries. Although medical costs increased, appropriations did not, with funding decreasing from $5,088,170 to $5,085,965 between 1940 and 1947. With funding for trachoma research and treatment curtailed, the prevalence of the disease increased in some parts of Indian Country, primarily among the elderly. Despite medical advances in the treatment and control of the disease, trachoma remained a highly prevalent communicable disease that plagued some Indian communities. By midcentury, trachoma ranked as one of the most prevalent diseases among American Indians.[23]

The Campaign against Tuberculosis

While the fight against trachoma was successful, the campaign against tuberculosis was less so. There was simply too much work and too few resources to eliminate the environmental contributors to the disease. Tuberculosis was a long-standing concern among American Indians that only grew worse. By the middle decades of the twentieth century, the incidence of tuberculosis remained excessive. Chippewa from the Bad River (Wisconsin) Reservation had neither a physician nor hospital services. Reverend W. H. Thompson, Pastor of the Methodist Church at Bad River, speculated that 80% of the funerals he conducted were related to tuberculosis. In the Southwest, the Navajo death rate was ten times the national average. In Montana, the chances of an Indian dying from tuberculosis were nine times greater than the general population. But nowhere was the rate higher than in Alaska, where the Alaska Native death rate was fourteen times the national average. This exceptional rate was attributed to poverty and neglect, although critic Haven Emerson believed it was the "direct and tragic result of political parsimony and general indifference" on the part of Congress.[24]

Tuberculosis was the most serious disease facing Indians. Scores of studies in Indian Country had demonstrated that. In 1935, Collier noted twenty-six different Indian health surveys indicated that 51,635 of the roughly 300,000 American Indians in the nation were treated for tuberculosis in a hospital, sanitaria or school infirmary. Little headway was made in combating the disease until 1935, when the BCG vaccination began.[25]

Prior to the introduction of the BCG, the standard treatment of tuberculosis was institutional care designed mostly for Indian children attending boarding schools; adults with tuberculosis were left to fend for themselves. While Commissioner William Jones ordered all infected children out of the schools and returned home, in 1904, many simply returned to the reservation and faced a slow death. In 1906, Congress authorized Leupp to tabulate the prevalence of the disease and provide an estimate of the cost needed to construct a tuberculosis sanitarium.

The construction of a sanitarium school in Phoenix, in 1909, was a start but did not provide care for all tubercular Indians. Within the next three years, the Indian Service opened four additional sanitaria, one each in Fort Lapwai, Idaho; Toledo, Iowa; Laguna, New Mexico; and Salem, Oregon. By 1912, the Indian tuberculosis incidence rate of 35.4 per 1,000 was three times the non-Indian rate of 12.1 per 1,000.[26]

John Collier extended an invitation to the scientific community to partner with the Indian medical service in the campaign against tuberculosis. In 1934, Townsend appointed Dr. Joseph D. Aronson, director of the Phipps Institute at the University of Pennsylvania, as chief medical researcher of the Indian Service. Aronson's task was to evaluate treatments for tuberculosis. Stationed in Albuquerque, New Mexico, and assisted by Dr. Esmond R. Long, Aronson implemented a tuberculosis program in which he vaccinated with BCG a number of Indians who tested negative to the tuberculin skin test. The BCG vaccine, first used to inoculate humans with the tuberculin virus in 1921, was thought to produce immunity to the disease. Among the first recipients of the BCG were several hundred school-aged children from the Pima Agency in Arizona.[27]

In the two years between February 1936 and February 1938, 1,565 Indian children under the age of nineteen (from five Indian agencies) were administered the BCG vaccine. A control group of 1,460 children of the same age was also established. All of the children tested negative to the skin test prior to the commencement of the study. Annual checkups included a skin test and x-ray. The preliminary results of the vaccination progress were encouraging. Among the vaccinated group there was one death from tuberculosis, while there were seventeen from the control group. The percentage of non-tubercular deaths was proportional in both groups. Although optimistic, Townsend remained cautious in declaring the preventive measure effective. Only time and additional research could validate the findings. Reminding Indian Service physicians to remain cautious, Townsend added, "The vaccine should be continued at least five more years, preferably ten. We will then have knowledge of its value when the child reaches the tuberculosis age and of how long it will be effective. Further studies relating to the differences in tribal responses to tuberculosis infection will be concomitant with the vaccine program and may reveal knowledge of everlasting importance."[28]

The results of the initial BCG vaccination program were reviewed in 1946, ten years after the process began. An analysis indicated that four of the 1,565 vaccinated children had died of tuberculosis versus twenty-eight of the 1,460 children in the control group. Although showing the vaccination reduced the mortality rate, the longitudinal study did not demonstrate that those treated remained free of the disease. Those who were vaccinated, however, were more likely to escape the disease.[29]

When the initial study was concluded in 1949, fourteen years after its inception, Fred Foard, assigned as medical director that year, concluded that BCG vaccinations were successful and ordered vaccinations of all Indian children testing negative to the tuberculin skin test. Among the first sites visited were Alaska Native villages and the Navajo and Hopi reservations in Arizona, where the disease was especially prevalent. These sites were selected not only because of their high incidence rates but also because they had been surveyed a year earlier, providing Foard with benchmark data. By the summer of 1949, 192 Indian schools were visited with 180 student populations completely vaccinated. Of the 17,000 children given the tuberculin skin test, 6,000 tested negative and received the BCG vaccine. The vaccination program was expanded, in 1952, when the Indian health program began vaccinating newborn babies—with the consent of the parents—after research indicated unvaccinated children were seven times more likely to contract tuberculosis than those who had been vaccinated.[30]

Despite the appearance of success in Indian Country, the effects of the BCG vaccine were not unanimously supported by all experts, some of whom argued a natural immunity to the tubercle bacillus was building up among the Indians. Townsend, for example, argued Indians were not predisposed to tuberculosis. "The Indians are developing a natural immunity, as in many of the x-ray films examined there is evidence of active lesions that have healed spontaneously without medical interference and without the Indian's knowledge that the disease had been existent." A 1954 study seemed to confirm the observation of Townsend, when Aronson concluded there was no "direct evidence that the B.C.G. vaccination was a contributing factor in reducing tuberculin infection." Although evidence as to why the incidence rate was declining was inconclusive, the fact remained that it was, as shown in Table 11.[31]

Table 11

Tuberculin Reactions among Unselected
and Non-BCG Vaccinated Indians in 1936-1941 and 1954

Age Group	No. Tested 1936-1941	Percentage* Positive	No. Tested 1954	Percentage* Positive	Percent Decline
5-9	2,167	31.3%	1,294	11.7%	62.6%
10-14	2,287	57.0%	936	23.5%	58.8%
15-19	1,300	81.0%	272	43.0%	46.9%

(* .00002 mg of Purified Protein Derivative Tuberculin)

(Source: The Trend of Tuberculosis Among Some Indian Tribes, 1955)

New Approaches to Treating Tuberculosis

Tuberculosis was attacked from other directions. In 1939, the Phipps Institute held a tuberculosis institute in Shawnee, Oklahoma, to disseminate information on the progress made in tubercular research. The Institute also conducted annual training for physicians and nurses to become tuberculosis specialists. Such training fostered the exchange of information regarding the most up-to-date procedures and, since the Indian Service lacked facilities to examine and interpret the many thousands of x-rays taken each year, tubercular x-rays were sent to the Phipps Institute where Indian Service physicians and nurses assisted in examining the photos, adding to their training.[32]

Widespread use of x-ray machines, used to detect incipient cases of tuberculosis, was implemented in 1937, when the first machine in Indian Country was put into service among the Lakota Sioux on the Pine Ridge (South Dakota) Reservation. After World War Two, the Indian Service purchased two mobile x-ray units to put into the field, with a third later added and assigned to the Navajo Reservation, where, in 1948, the tuberculosis death rate was 302.4 per thousand, compared with 33.4 for the general population. The mobile units were particularly beneficial in that x-rays could be developed and read in the field rather than sending it to Pennsylvania, although the fact that there were just three units limited their overall effectiveness.[33]

After 1952, the Indian Service entered into cooperative projects with Cornell University Medical Center for the treatment of tubercular patients. The joint effort was instrumental in treating tubercular patients with isoniazid, the first drug used to effectively treat tuberculosis. In 1953, Cornell provided a surgeon and a chest specialist for the Indian Service hospital at Fort Defiance and began a long-term project designed to elevate the health of the Navajo in a culturally sensitive manner. In addition to treating Navajos, the specialists trained Indian Service physicians in the treatment of tuberculosis, with the Indian Service assigning many of its physicians to the Fort Defiance hospital for brief periods of training.

Congressional Parsimony

The medical breakthroughs and new forms of treatment were welcomed additions to the Division of Indian Health. But rather than support the efforts of the Indian Service, Congress under funded the program. Indian Commissioner John Nichols requested $11,000,000 to fight tuberculosis in 1949, with Congress granting him $2,400,000. The results were expected. The Indian health program accommodated only half of all American Indians and Alaska Natives with active cases of tuberculosis. Lacking hospital facilities and field services, Medical Director Fred Foard argued many Indians would be compelled to "wander at large among their own people, each a definite danger to those [with] whom he comes into contact." Even where hospitals were available, exiguous funding meant just six in ten beds were available, in 1948. By 1949, the Indian Service tuberculosis sanitaria, including all contract facilities, accommodated an average of 592 patients, or just

63% of operating capacity. The under utilization rate was attributed to Congressional parsimony.[34]

With insufficient funding, the spread of tuberculosis—although slowed—could not be prevented in Indian Country due to the unavailability of hospital accommodations and preventive care. Reductions in funding also meant contractual services with state and local governments lapsed. At the Minnesota Chippewa Agency, insufficient funds required twenty-eight tubercular Indians be dismissed from the state sanitarium and returned to their homes—all a "possible source of infection" to those with whom they came into contact.[35]

As midcentury arrived, the Division of Indian Health boasted of advances in the campaign against tuberculosis. Nonetheless, tuberculosis remained the major hindrance to an acceptable standard of Indian healthcare as seen by two yardsticks. First, nearly 40% of the Indian health budget was spent on tuberculosis control and treatment, representing an enormous expense of time and energy in trying to deal with the effects of the disease. Secondly, although the Indian tuberculosis mortality rate declined proportionately with non-Indians, the 1953 American Indian and Alaska Native rate was still higher than the non-Indian rate for 1935, as Table 12 indicates. Indian health status remained two decades behind that of the general population.[36]

Table 12
Mortality Rates for Tuberculosis: Select Years 1900-1954
(Per 100,000 Population)

Year	Indian	All Races
1900	N/A	194.4
1905	N/A	179.9
1910	N/A	153.8
1915	N/A	140.1
1920	N/A	113.1
1925	N/A	84.8
1930	N/A	71.1
1935	278.6	55.1
1940	240.2	45.9
1945	200.8	39.9
1950	121.1	22.5
1954	49.1	10.2

(Source: Public Health Service, 1957)

A Reality Check

If the Division of Indian Health needed a dose of reality by which to measure the effects of budget cut backs and Congressional parsimony, it need look no further than the Navajo Nation. Sprawled over 15,000,000 acres of land in Arizona, New Mexico and Utah, nearly 70,000 Navajos lived with one of the highest mortality rates in the United States. Some medical experts likened Navajo health challenges to those of the United States a century earlier. Tuberculosis and trachoma remained widespread. Infant mortality was four times greater among the Navajo than the nation at-large and pneumonia, gastritis, enteritis and colitis were twenty times higher. The challenges facing the Navajo were, with few exceptions, little different than those facing non-Indians except in degree, something attributed to "environmental conditions, want of education and adequate medical care."[37]

While the obstacles seemed great they were surmountable, even if they were "a commanding challenge." To alleviate the assortment of health complications, the American Medical Association threw its weight behind a proposal to construct a medical center within the Navajo Nation with the capacity of serving as a clearinghouse for all diagnostic, medical and surgical matters. Such a facility required an expert medical and surgical staff. To retain specialists at the medical center, the American Medical Association encouraged the Indian Service to set up a rotating medical service and staff the following specialists: Internal medicine, general surgery, pediatrics, obstetrics, thoracic surgeon, orthopedics, ophthalmologist, dermatologist, neuropsychiatrist, pathologist, roentgenologist, and various laboratory specialists.[38]

The Navajo Nation was not the only tribal nation facing serious health challenges. In 1947, Commissioner William Brophy toured Alaska to see the challenges facing Alaska Natives. While witnessing firsthand the devastating effects of tuberculosis, Brophy contracted pneumonia and then developed tuberculosis. Before leaving, he noted Alaska Natives needed a wide gamut of supplies to fight tuberculosis. Although Congress might appropriate funds for hospital, sanitarium and tuberculosis equipment, the Commissioner argued facilities alone were not enough. The severity of Alaska Native health struck a chord with Brophy, who sympathized with them. "The siege has dramatically brought home to me the necessity that we increase our assault on all fronts, the medical, educational, economic and social."

Brophy resigned as Indian commissioner, in 1949, and—especially after John Nichols resigned a year later—Congress assumed control of the Indian Service and scaled back funding and services further. President Harry Truman's "Fair Deal" sought integration of all Americans into American society. To do this, Congress sought national conformity. Indian programs were slashed and the termination of the federal-Indian relationship began. In the process, Congress renewed its interest in consolidating the Indian medical service with the Public Health Service.[39]

Notes

1. Robert Gessner, *Massacre: A Survey of Today's American Indian* (New York: Jonathan Cape and Harrison Smith, 1931), 255-256, 260.

2. Donald L. Fixico, *Termination and Relocation: Federal Indian Policy, 1945-1960* (Albuquerque: University of New Mexico Press, 1986), 35, 46. Most of the proposed closures were in Oklahoma.

3. Paul de Kruif, "They Wait for Light," *Country Gentleman* (September 1940), in Rosella Sanders, "Indian Medical Service Pioneers in Trachoma Treatment," *Indians at Work* (8:4, December 1940), 32-33.

4. *Contagious and Infectious Disease among the Indians*, 19-40. J.G. Townsend, "Trachoma, Dreaded Eye Disease, Being Conquered," *Indian at Work* (7:4, December 1939), 11. "Observations on Indian Health Problems and Facilities," 41 (appendix A).

5. *Health Services for American Indians* (Washington, DC: GPO, Department of Health, Education and Welfare, Public Health Service, 1957), 57. Spain introduced trachoma to the American Indians in the sixteenth century, possibly with the settlement of Santa Fe by Juan de Oñate. Early American trappers and traders, as well as other European explorers, never specifically referred to trachoma but did frequently mention "bad eyes," "sore eyes" or "scrofulous eyes," all references to trachoma. The term trachoma was not used in connection with American Indians until after the turn of the twentieth century. "Trachoma in Certain Indian Schools," *Senate Report no. 1025*, 60th Congress, 2nd session, 2. Townsend, "Trachoma, Dreaded Eye Disease, Being Conquered," 8-11.

6. "An Act for the investigation, treatment, and prevention of trachoma among the Indians," 35 Stat. 642.

7. Meriam, 210.

8. Fox, 1544-1545. In four village or school sites, Fox found 351 cases of trachoma out of 1,168 individuals. Fox argued, "There is no good reason why the Indians should be permitted to go blind in the presence of known methods of prevention." *Board of Indian Commissioners Annual Report*, 1925, 14-15.

9. Meriam, 212-213; Gessner 219.

10. Meriam, 11.

11. P. Thygeson and F.I. Proctor, "Filterability of Trachoma virus," *Archives of Ophthalmology* (13, 1930), 1018. P. Thygeson, F.I. Proctor and P. Richards, "Etiologic significance of the elementary body in trachoma," *American Journal of Ophthalmology* (18, 1935), 811. L.A. Julianelle, M.C. Morris and R.W. Harrison, "Studies on the infectivity of trachoma: Further observations on the filterability of the infectious agent," *American Journal of Ophthalmology* (20, 1937), 890.

12. Wesley G. Forster, "Trachoma," *American Journal of Ophthalmology* (27:10, October 1944), 1107-1117. *Annual Report*, 1937, 237. "Nature of Filtrable Agent of Trachoma," *Journal of the American Medical Association* (111:20, November 12, 1938), 1879. Thygeson and Richards made their conclusion based on twenty-two filtration experiments on a human volunteer and monkeys and baboons.

13. Williams studied the hemoglobinophilic bacillus, which she isolated from the cases of papillary trachoma in which these bodies or inclusions were present. She concluded that the bacillus and inclusion were probably the same in papillary trachoma and, hence, the bacillus was probably the cause of trachoma. *Contagious and Infectious Diseases among the Indians*, 17.

14. Sanders, 33. Shortly after being healed of trachoma, Brown was killed in an automobile accident. Thygeson called Brown a "good soldier throughout." *Annual Report*, 1938, 239. "Nature of Filtrable Agent of Trachoma."

15. Four physicians were appointed to the committee at the salary of $1 a year: Harry S. Gradle, Lawrence T. Post, William L. Benedict and Louis S. Greene. Their first meeting was November 10, 1937, in Washington, D.C. Townsend, "Special Trachoma Advisory Committee holds first Meeting," *Indians at Work* (4:6, December 1, 1937), 32. Townsend, "Trachoma, Dreaded Eye Disease, Being Conquered," 8.

16. Sanders, 33.

17. Fred Loe, "Sulfanilamide Treatment of Trachoma," *Journal of the American Medical Association* (111:15, October 8, 1938), 1371-1372. Loe gives a brief history of both patients. "Lifting the Shadows," *Indians at Work* (8:9, May 1941), 11-13.

18. Townsend, "Trachoma, Dreaded Eye Disease, Being Conquered," 9.

19. Loe, "Sulfanilamide Treatment of Trachoma," 1371. There was also considerable paling of the conjunctiva and a flattening of the granules and follicles, although it took several months for this to occur. The granules of the lower eyelids were the last objective symptoms to disappear. Dr. Harry S. Gradle, "Abstract of Discussion," *Journal of the American Medical Association* (111:15, October 8, 1938), 1372. Wesley Forster, "Treatment of Trachoma," *American Journal of Ophthalmology* (23:5, May 1940). Phillips Thygeson, "The Treatment of Trachoma," *American Journal of Ophthalmology* (23:6, June 1940).

20. *Annual Report*, 1939, 47. Studies were conducted in Arizona, Minnesota, Oregon, Montana, New Mexico, Wyoming and Nevada, as well as at the Fort Apache Trachoma School. "Medical News," *Journal of the American Medical Association* (113:13, September 23, 1939), 1233. Among the Navajo the tests ran from June 1 to July 17. Townsend, "Trachoma, Dreaded Eye Disease, Being Conquered," 9-10.

21. *Annual Report*, 1939, 47. Townsend, 9-10. Townsend compared the record at Fort Apache to the pre-sulfanilamide treatment days, when only 215 of the 428 children had the disease arrested (thirty-seven in 1936; sixty-five in 1937; sixty-seven in 1938; and forty-six in 1939). The experiment at Ft. Apache lasted five years. The first year had all cases treated alike with a 2% solution of silver nitrate applied to the conjunctiva three times a week, followed by irrigation with boric acid. During the second and third years treatment was altered according to type and severity of the disease. The 2% silver nitrate treatment was continued and daily chaulmoogra oil massages were added. The fourth year saw the introduction of mineral oil instead of chaulmoogra oil. The final year sulfanilamide was used exclusively.

22. *Annual Report*, 1943, 281. "Health Program of Indian Service," 33-34. In the former, the rate of decrease is shown as 30% to 5%. The Warm Springs program was as much educational as it was medical. "Lifting the Shadows," 11-14.

23. "Trachoma Eradication," *Science* (90:2341, February 15, 1939), Supple-

ment 10. "Lifting the Shadows," 13. In 1939, Dr. R. Siri, a Siamese physician visiting the United States on a Rockefeller grant, examined the sulfanilamide treatment developed by the Indian Service for use in his home country of Siam, where 20% of the country's 15,000,000 people were afflicted with the disease. Trachoma treatment, once based on guesswork, had become relatively pain free and effective by the 1940s.

24. Emerson, 219. The Bad River agency farmer was reportedly dispensing drugs to the Indians. When asked about why he did so, the farmer responded, "It is simple to treat the Indians." Gessner, 208.

25. Meriam, 204. "Tuberculosis among Indians," *Indians at Work* (3:8, December 1, 1935), 35. There were fourteen tuberculosis sanitaria and seventy-nine regular hospitals serving the Indian population.

26. Gregg, 15. Education Circular no. 106, March 23, 1904. 34 Stat. 328. *Contagious and Infectious Disease among the Indians*, 41-44.

27. Leon Albert Calmette and his assistant Camette Guerin at the Louis Pasteur Institute in France derived the BCG vaccine from a strain of mycobacterium bovis that was attenuated. "Dr. Joseph David Aronson appointed Special Expert on Tuberculosis," *Journal of the American Medical Association* (105:14, October 5, 1935), 1125. Long was appointed as a Special Consultant after conducting a tuberculosis survey among the Papago of Arizona, in 1933. "Community Meeting on Health Problems at the New Salt River Day School, Arizona," *Indians at Work* (3:24, August 1, 1936), 13-14. Aronson explained the principles of tuberculosis via x-ray pictures and microscopic slides to several hundred Pimas from the Salt River Pima-Maricopa Indian Reservation.

28. Joseph D. Aronson, "Appraisal of Protective Value of BCG Vaccine," *Journal of the American Medical Association* (149:4, May 24, 1952), 334-343. Aronson concluded, "The evidence for the development of original resistance following primary infection with tubercle bacilli is sound." The test group included individuals from the Pima, Wind River, Turtle Mountain and Rosebud Agencies as well as the Tlingit, Haida and Tsimshian in southeastern Alaska. *Annual Report*, 1939, 47. Townsend, "Indian Health—Past, Present and Future," 38.

29. *Annual Report*, 1946, 362.

30. "A.M.A. Leaders and Secretary Krug Plan New Medical Missions," *Journal of the American Medical Association* (139:14, April 2, 1949), 927. The new mission of the Division of Indian Health was to focus on medical care and advanced instruction for Indian Service physicians. Sitka, Alaska was targeted as the first site. *Annual Report*, 1949. Eight medical teams in Arizona, Colorado, New Mexico, Utah, Idaho, Montana, Nebraska, North Dakota, South Dakota and Wyoming provided vaccinations.

31. Townsend, "Indian Health—Past, Present and Future," 35. Joseph D. Aronson and Helen C. Taylor, "The Trend of Tuberculosis Infections among some Indian Tribes and the Effectiveness of BCG Vaccination on Tuberculin Testing," *The American Review of Tuberculosis and Pulmonary Disease* (The National Tuberculosis Association, 72, July-December 1955), 49.

32. In 1940, the Public Health Service assigned Dr. Horace DeLien to the Indian Service for tuberculosis control among the Indians of California, Utah and Nevada. "Medical News," *Journal of the American Medical Association* (115:11, September 14,

1940), 1870. Townsend, "The Battle against Tuberculosis Goes Forward," *Indian at Work* (6:8, April 1934), 35. There were seventy-three attendees at the third annual institute in 1939. The purpose was to familiarize physicians and nurses with the standard household and community phases of the tuberculosis problem.

33. In 1939, Loe surveyed the Rosebud Reservation, taking more than 2,000 x-rays. Because Rosebud had a tribal community health program, any Sioux released from a sanitarium had a letter sent home warning the community of the potential health risk and offering an examination and x-ray. Mary McKay, "The Rosebud Sioux Organize for Health," 8. In April 1951, the University of Utah medical school entered into a contractual arrangement with the Navajo Nation to serve as medical advisors. In March of that same year, the Association on American Indian Affairs, Inc., announced the appointment of a national medical committee to work for the immediate improvement of the conditions affecting the tribe. Emerson, "Indian Health—Victim of Neglect," 219. Foard, "The Health of the American Indians," 1404.

34. Foard, "Health Facilities for Indians," 329.

35. W.F. Braasch, B.J. Branton and A.J. Chesley, "Survey of Medical Care Among the Upper Midwest Indians," *Journal of the American Medical Association* (139:4, 1949), 224.

36. This is based on fiscal year 1956. *Health Services for American Indians*, 41, 128.

37. John Adair, Kurt Deuschle and Walsh McDermott, "Patterns of Health and Disease Among the Navahos," *The Annals of the American Academy of Political and Social Science* (311, May 1957), 80-94. Lewis Moorman, "Health of the Navajo-Hopi Indians," *Journal of the American Medical Association* (139:6, February 5, 1949), 370-375. Syphilis, diarrhea, dental decay and congenital disorders were also widespread. On the other hand, the Navajo were virtually free of cancer, diabetes and arteriosclerosis. Faulty nutrition, physical hardships, overcrowded hogans, remoteness, language barriers, religious beliefs, lack of effective case finding, poor management and lack of sanitarium care and follow-up care were blamed for the poor health status of the Navajo.

38. In 1937 the Navajo had received a new $450,000 hospital at Fort DeFiance, with the old hospital being converted into a tuberculosis sanitarium. "Medical News," *Journal of the American Medical Association* (109:13, September 25, 1937).

39. Fixico, 33, 37.

CHAPTER SIX

A Justified Wave of Criticism?

In the 1920s, three American Indians arrived in Washington, DC, and toured the offices of the Indian Service. The three men sat attentively as Indian Service officials explained the plans of the government to provide them with the best medical care possible. "Won't this be great for your people," one official stated? "Won't these plans make them healthy?" The leader of the delegation gazed out the window upon the sites of Washington. Turning away from the window, he quietly stated, "Heap big wind. No rain."[1]

While stereotypic, the statement illustrated American Indians were both skeptical and cynical. Assured an equal chance to compete in American society, many American Indians and Alaska Natives were too ill to do so. Reductions in the number of medical personnel and funding during World War Two compounded matters. While there were improvements in some areas, mortality rates remained high. The inescapable fact was American Indians were at a nadir. Medical advances benefiting the United States only peripherally reached Indian Country. Medical science, which found new ways to treat, cure and eliminate disease and extend life expectancy among non-Indians (especially in urban areas), rarely reached Indians.[2]

The Challenges of Service-Oriented Medical Care

Although the Indian Service was constrained by political considerations to make do with limited resources and less-than-desirably-trained personnel, it frequently blamed the Indians for its deficiencies. In 1955, Indian Commissioner Glenn Emmons placed culpability for the difficulties of the medical program at the feet of the "rural, isolated, culturally different and economically depressed" Indians it served. While there was an element of truth to Emmons' assertion (and applicable in some respects to all of rural America), such comments ignored the need for better services.

Isolated Indian Service facilities made staffing difficult and there remained a number of reservations without health services or physicians. At the Fort Berthold (North Dakota) Reservation, for example, the nearest doctor was twenty-eight miles away and the nearest government hospital 125 miles away. The Forest County (Wisconsin) Pottawatomie had no hospital. When Congressman George Schneider (R-WI) introduced a bill to authorize $125,000 to construct an Indian hospital in the county, in 1929, the Indian Service opposed it, killing the bill in committee. Private practice physician George H. Reddick of nearby Wabeno, Wisconsin, suggested the Indian Service opposed the bill because it didn't "want to do anything for the Indian."[3]

Already spread thin, additional Indian Service facilities required additional staffing, which meant appropriations would either have to increase or they would have to be taken from existing facilities. At the same time, reports of ineptness and contempt on the part of Indian Service physicians abounded. In Wisconsin, it was alleged Indian Service contract physician E. G. Ovitz refused to attend to a pregnant woman who subsequently gave birth at home where the baby "dropped out on the floor—dead." Another Indian woman hemorrhaged to death because Ovitz refused to see her. A nineteen-year-old Indian man suffering with a 103-degree fever, labored breathing and pleurisy with effusion, was simply ignored by Ovitz. When a nearby private practice physician informed the young man's father to seek immediate medical attention for his son, Ovitz refused to treat him because "a private practitioner had informed him that the case was serious." Four days later, the father arrived at the home of the private practice physician begging him to do something for his son. The young man died of tuberculosis four months later without the Indian Service physician ever seeing him.[4]

In 1929, other stories of incompetence and challenges to service-oriented care came to light. A contract physician working among the Bad River Chippewa in northern Wisconsin refused to serve any Indian patient who could not pay for services. Dr. H. G. Mertens, a private practice physician near the Red Cliff (Wisconsin) Chippewa Reservation, noted the Indians had been without medical care for years. While there was a contract physician that visited the reservation one afternoon a week, if the Indians "did not come on the day set aside for them" they were not treated. Magpie Smith, a Winnebago from Nebraska, shared how her daughter had been badly burned. While the government physician came and looked at the daughter, he did nothing to help her. A local Catholic mission assisted Smith in dressing her daughter's burns. The Indian Service physician did not return until the child was dying a month later. When an elderly Winnebago woman injured her knee, she visited the agency hospital where she was bed-ridden for two months, growing weaker each day. In desperation, the woman's daughter procured funds to transport her mother to a hospital in Sioux City, Iowa, where she underwent surgery. Without her knowledge or consent, the elderly woman was returned to the agency hospital where her leg was amputated. She died nine hours later.[5]

Another Indian Service physician refused to treat a woman who died of spasms in childbirth because he was allegedly unwilling "to face the situation [as] he was about to receive his transfer." When Florence S. Sanford of Berkley, California, visited northern Arizona to observe the status of the Navajo, she was appalled at the level of sickness and the overall conditions she encountered. When she inquired of a local Indian trader named Zoarl Styles why he did not report the agency physician who refused to treat two women with sick babies, the trader explained "he couldn't report it because . . . the agent would take it out on him." In northern California, an Indian Service physician delayed three years in performing cataract surgery (without anesthetic) on a Hoopa man, who for all his pain and suffering received only partial restoration of his sight.[6]

When Senator William Pine (R-OK) inquired of Dr. Warren C. Hunt whether Indian Service physicians took a genuine interest in their work and if they did all they could to help the Indians, Hunt admitted there were "real shortcomings" within the Indian medical service, with some physicians showing concern and others not. Not surprisingly, some Indians exhibited an intense dislike of government physicians. Herbert Edwards of the Meriam study, linked service utilization on the part of the Indians with service-driven care on the part of disinterested physicians. "[M]ore Indians would accept the services of physicians," Edwards opined, "if their interests were solicited."[7]

The Indians' aversion of Indian Service physicians was influenced by the whirlwind campaign against trachoma when a "reign of terror (i.e., tarsectomies) swept through the Indian Country." Cultural challenges compounded matters, especially among traditional American Indians. Opening Indian Service facilities to non-Indians added to the challenges. Non-Indian residents of Lander, Wyoming, refused to utilize the Indian hospital on the Wind River Reservation. Conversely, the Rosebud Sioux did not want non-Indians utilizing their facility. Such intransigent attitudes compounded cultural issues.[8]

Socio-economic factors were important participants in the medical discussion of the American Indians and Alaska Natives. Considering these indices, it is staggering that American Indians and Alaska Natives *were as well as they were*. Houses were inadequate, poorly ventilated and overcrowded. Sanitary conditions were completely wanting. Overall educational achievement was low, leading the American Medical Association to couple economic dependence with alcoholism, illegitimacy and poor social and sanitary conditions. Some vocal critics argued that if the American people knew the true conditions in Indian Country "a justified wave of criticism would sweep the country."[9]

Lacking a full understanding of what it was facing, the Indian health program struggled to make progress in the overall campaign against disease.

Accurate medical statistics and analysis were non-existent prior to 1940. More than one-third of Indian births were unregistered in 1940, with causes of death remaining educated guesses or based on the hearsay of agency personnel. Important differences in the age-sex composition of American Indians and non-Indians existed, with Indians having a much higher percentage of youth than other Americans. Although the high Indian infant mortality rate partially compensated for this, the large number of young Indians in age groups with low death rates had a depressing effect on the overall crude Indian death rate. The Indian death rate from diarrhea and enteritis remained eight times the national rate. The infant mortality rate was four times greater and pneumonia, which had almost been eliminated as a major killer in the general population, still struck Indian Country three times the national average. Studies among the Pueblos of New Mexico found the incidence of amebic dysentery was "extremely high." Some of the Pueblos experienced a 40% incidence rate, twice the national rate. A study among Alaska Natives in the lower Kuskokwin region revealed an alarming spread of meningitis. The combined efforts of the Division of Indian Health and the Alaska Territorial Health Department placed the cause of the disease on the presence of dental caries occasioned by the use of refined sugar. Overall progress in mitigating poor health was limited, and health parity with non-Indians remained illusive.[10]

Childhood Diseases

It had long been federal Indian policy to focus efforts on the children, a generation upon whom the Indian Service placed great hope and faith each year. In 1934, in an effort to increase its commitment to children, John Collier initiated a survey of Indian Country to determine the prevalence of congenital disorders. Although surveying only a fraction of Indian Country, the study found 770 children suffering from bone deformities, mostly the result of congenital hip dislocations and tuberculosis. While a few physicians took steps to provide treatment for children, the Indian Service largely ignored congenital disorders, focusing on the more dramatic maladies such as tuberculosis and trachoma. When Congress enacted into law the Social Security Act of 1935, it required states to provide services for all crippled children, including American Indian and Alaska Native, or face the loss of federal grants-in-aid. Arizona and New Mexico elected to forfeit federal aid rather than provide services for Indian children, basing their decisions on the Indians' ward (and non-tax-paying) status and their state organic acts, which denied Indian wards services from the state.[11]

Despite a growing number of state and county facilities providing children's services, many Indians were unable to avail themselves of such treatment due to the distance such facilities were from their homes. By midcentury, for example, 145 counties provided services for crippled children. Yet, this covered just 60% of the Indian population. Of this number, only one-third of American Indians had access to such treatment. In order to obtain services, it was common for children to travel 100 miles or more. In many cases—especially in the West—the only transportation available was a wagon drawn by a team of horses, making travel slow and arduous. Three years after its first survey of congenital disorders, the Indian Service established a preventorium for underweight children among the Spirit Lake Dakota on the Ft. Totten (North Dakota) Reservation, where specialized care and treatment were available to diagnose tubercular and other childhood infections. Its distance from other Indian reservations, however, limited its overall impact in Indian Country.[12]

The lack of pediatricians and nutritionists in the Indian Service was more of a difficulty, considering infant and childhood diseases were among the principle causes of death. The Superintendent of the Papago (Tohono O'odham) Reservation reported the population curve of the tribe resembled that of medieval Europe. "Of approximately 260 infants born each year, one-fourth die within twelve months; at the age of 6 there are only 160 left; at the age of eighteen only 125." The life expectancy of non-Indian infants was sixty years in 1949, while that of Papago infants was seventeen. "The comparison of the weighted Papago age curve with that of the United States as a whole," medical director Fred Foard concluded, "tells an almost incredible health story. Only a birth rate double that of the country as a whole enables the Papagos to survive at all."[13]

Despite some additions to infant and early childhood care and treatment, Indian children still faced a variety of challenges. Chicken pox, impetigo, measles, whooping cough, infant paralysis and sundry health complications were more prevalent among Indian children than among non-Indian children. In 1954, American Indians faced a measles death rate twenty times the non-Indian rate. Deaths from pneumonia and influenza were four times the non-Indian rate and infant deaths were three times the comparable non-Indian rate. Maternal mortality rates were substantially higher among American Indians, as seen in Table 13.[14]

Table 13

Infant and Maternal Mortality Rates:
Select Years, 1940-1953

Year	Maternal Deaths	Per 1,000 Live Births	U.S. All	Infant Births	Infant Deaths	Per 1,000 Live Births	U.S. All
1940	69	7.2	3.8	9,547	1,077	112.8	47.0
1945	57	5.6	2.1	10,172	N/A	N/A	38.3
1950	35	2.6	0.6	13,362	1,097	82.1	29.2
1953	29	1.9	0.6	14,932	1,136	76.1	27.8

(Source: *Health Services For American Indians*, 1957)

Dietary Deficiencies

Many of the infant and childhood diseases were exacerbated by dietary changes or poor diets. Physicians frequently commented on the severity of intestinal diseases among Indian children, which they attributed to poor diets. The American Medical Association suggested a high illegitimacy rate was a sociological threat to Indian children. Many of these children lived in overcrowded homes that increased the likelihood of disease. Lacking a formal education, some of these mothers provided unhealthy food to their infants after they left the breast. Cheyenne mothers were known to give crying infants bottles filled with coffee or tea. Pueblo mothers fed their infants chili, beans, green fruits and melons. Some Sioux mothers gave red meat to their infant children.[15]

Malnutrition overwhelmed the Indian Service in its effort to mitigate infant diseases. "The Indians in the continental United States and the natives of Alaska have undergone marked changes in dietary habits during the last two generations," Collier wrote in 1944. "The introduction of processed foods through schools, hospitals, and trading posts has meant too often the discarding of native foods, rich in essential vitamins." The introduction and heavy reliance upon processed white flour, refined sugar, canned goods, and other government commodities combined with the exclusion of traditional foods "resulted in poor nutrition, undernourishment, dental defects and susceptibility to disease."[16]

When field nurse Eleanor B. Jones joined the Indian Service in 1927, she expected to serve as a field nurse conducting home visits and reporting on what could be done to improve the state of health among the Navajo. Assigned instead to Tuba City Indian School, Jones witnessed widespread malnutrition with the government physician turning a deaf ear on the matter. While there was "a dispensary stacked full of chemicals of various kinds," Jones noted, they "did not appear to have ever been used." Jones was so repulsed by the lack of concern at the agency level that she resigned the Indian Service less than a month later. In Wisconsin, the challenge was glaringly brought to the public's attention. A twenty-five-month-old infant was examined by private practice physician R.L. Frisbie of Rhinelander, Wisconsin, and found to weigh thirteen pounds. Just twenty-six inches in length, the child crawled, but did not walk and mumbled, but did not speak."[17]

In an effort to combat dietary challenges, Collier in 1940 assigned a full-time physician to study the food habits of Southwestern tribal nations. The physician concluded foods were "markedly deficient in certain nutritive values." To overcome this deficiency, studies using bean sprouts as a source of nutrients were instituted among the Tohono O'odham Nation (Papago). Among several Pueblo villages, ponds were constructed to employ fish as a nutritional supplement. Although the overall extent of nutritional deficiencies was unknown, the Public Health Service opined a rapidly changing Indian way of life led to a diet lacking protein and iron, which complicated the healthy development of prenatal women and their unborn babies. Among prenatal mothers, anemia and obesity resulted, while among infants, poor musculature development and anemia were present. Despite the growing evidence of malnutrition, nutritionists were not permanently added to the Division of Indian Health, although one was assigned to the Navajo Nation. To alleviate the effects of malnutrition, the Public Health Service encouraged Congress to appropriate funds for the appointment of at least one "well-trained nutrition consultant" for each Indian agency.[18]

In the interim, new medical studies made public poor health conditions among American Indians and Alaska Natives. A 1949 study of Hopi and Navajo nutritional status concluded the Indians were doing "very well on a quite simple diet." Compared to non-Indians, the Navajo and Hopi were "virtually free from cancer and diabetes and they have a very low incidence rate of heart and blood-vessel disease (arteriosclerosis)." Non-Indian rates for these same conditions were rising. To a large degree the Indians were free of cancer and diabetes because they experienced a lower life expectancy than non-Indians. The authors of the study concluded the Indians were better off than non-Indians in these disease categories because of "the limited diet, the slow pace [of life], and the desert poise." The study prophetically concluded that the rate would increase "as we continue to give them . . . 'firewater,' soda pop, candy bars, and spearmint."[19]

Dental Services

Dietary changes affected the periodontal care of the Indians. Although there were more than fifty dentists in Indian Country by 1955, the services they provided related to extractions and emergency care. Already in 1936, the Public Health Service recognized Indian dental needs were at least equal to, but likely greater than, similar socio-economic groups. The introduction of high processed, sugar-laden foods after World War Two ensured tooth decay and increased the demand for dental care.[20]

Lacking funds and the professional expertise, the Indian Service relied on the Public Health Service for dental assistance. In 1932, when fewer than ten dentists served nearly a quarter of a million Indians, the Public Health Service detailed C.T. Messner to the Division of Indian Health to serve as the first Chief Dental Officer. Messner reorganized the dental program and increased its size to twenty-eight full-time and seventeen part-time dentists by 1939, although the isolation and rural nature of Indian Country was one factor in the episodic care provided. But isolation was not the core factor: most Indian agencies were visited by a dentist but once every other year—a preventive schedule not conducive to dental hygiene.

To his credit, Collier worked to overcome the obstacle of distance by initiating mobile dental clinics. Instituted on a trial basis among the Pueblos of

New Mexico in 1935, the clinics became permanent a year later when two additional "dental clinics on wheels" were placed in the field. Assigned to each was an American Indian trained to assist the dentist as well as drive and service the vehicle. Not all tribes were willing to patiently wait while the Division of Indian Health planned services. The Navajo Nation petitioned for, and received from Congress, $5,000 of their funds for the staffing of a dental unit, which they located in their new hospital at Fort Defiance. The funds were then replenished through the collection of dental fees.[21]

In 1950, in an effort to coordinate the scattered dental programs more effectively (and part of another general reorganization of the Indian Service), the chief dental officer was reassigned from Washington, DC, to Denver, Colorado. With headquarters in the West, the dental officer was in closer contact with the dental programs serving the Indians. More importantly, the move corresponded with a review of forty-six Indian agencies to determine the extent of dental caries among the Indians. Combined with an evaluation of the supply of dental and prophylactic services available, the reorganization gave credence to plans for dental expansion. To fill immediate needs, the Indian Service conducted a service-wide inventory to determine what supplies and equipment were necessary to improve dental care. Once this was quantified, the Indian Service—notoriously lacking funds—solicited discarded equipment from other government agencies, with the U.S. Navy supplying the bulk of it. The passage of the 1950 Doctor-Dentist Draft Law provided additional commissioned corps dentists to the understaffed Indian dental team via details from the Public Health Service.[22] A corollary initiative was inaugurated the following year when the Indian Service shifted its philosophy from providing emergency dental care to the conservation of Indian periodontics. The goal was to provide complete dental care for all Indian children under the age of nineteen.[23]

As part of its new approach, the Indian Service increasingly emphasized prevention by using topical fluoride applications, fluoridating communal water sources, reducing the intake of carbohydrates and instituting general dental hygiene. Although it looked good in theory, the new approach required additional funding and personnel, both of which were unlikely given the congressional push to terminate Indian programs after 1946. Despite a Congressional desire to withdraw services, the Public Health Service encouraged Congress to provide funding to more than double the number of full-time dentists from fifty-two to 130. This was essential to mitigate the backlog of demand. James Shaw, appointed director of the Indian health program in 1952, requested an annual budget of $3 million for dental services, to be implemented over a five-year span.[24]

Understanding the Cultural Side of Medicine

The creation of tribal health boards was an important component in the campaign on disease. Not only did such boards foster greater Indian acceptance of modern medical services but they also provided greater understanding of the tribal conception of well-being to health care workers. Working with federal health officials at the reservation level, such boards established and implemented programs designed to improve general health habits. They recommended health codes that fit the unique needs of the tribe and, if approved by the tribal council, had the force of law. In short, health boards served as models for implementing sound health practices among tribal members and helped mitigate many of the fears Indians had regarding Western medicine in general and non-Indian physicians and nurses in particular.[25]

Indian acceptance of Western medicine was both a result of, and a reason for, Indian health boards. General acceptance of modern medicine was perhaps the most significant health development among American Indians and Alaska Natives prior to 1950. Some American Indians recognized the value of modern medicine in their quest for good health, while others simply resigned themselves to the fact that it was a reality they could no longer avoid. Others—especially the more traditional Indians—continued to reject the "white man's medicine," as they viewed it as being in conflict with their cultural and religious beliefs. Many tribes, for instance, abandoned the house where a deceased relative had lived. As a result, there was great apprehension on the part of Indians in utilizing hospitals where death was a common occurrence.

Through a combination of factors, including health education for children, Indians overcame cultural barriers and recognized the benefits of modern medicine. An Indian mother giving birth with the aid of midwives could not be expected to suddenly give birth in a hospital among people she did not know. Centuries-old customs would not change over night. Only through Community health education—which tribal health boards facilitated—could such challenges be overcome. But traditional medicine was by no means discarded. Philosophically, most Indians believed health was symptomatic of a harmonious relationship between man and his environment. Health was associated with blessings and natural beauty, while illness was a sign that man had fallen out of harmony with his environment. Many Indians continued to hold such beliefs but recognized the role of modern medicine, as well. By the 1950s, an increasing number of American Indians utilized services provided by the Indian health program.[26]

Federal recognition of tribal shaman and medicine men during Collier's tenure played a role in reducing the apprehension of some Indians. Recognizing the legitimacy of tribal culture and medicinal practices went far in reducing cultural barriers, both among Indians and non-Indians. In 1940, Navajo medicine men were invited to participate in the dedication of two new Indian hospitals. As part of the dedication ceremony, the medicine men offered traditional prayers and blessings, lending credence to the Western institution. A reciprocal appreciation between traditional healers and modern physicians also opened the door to greater Indian utilization of medical services and reduced Indian apprehensions.[27]

Validation of community medicine was another important factor. Before the imposition of Western medicine, medicine men involved the tribal community in the healing process via sings or ceremonies. Since care within this system was given among families and within a familial environment, there was a psychotherapeutic aspect to healing. In 1949, Lewis Moorman led a team of specialists from the American Medical Association on a fact-finding tour among the Navajo and Hopi, concluding "though we question the efficacy of the medicine man's way of employing a few herbs and singing, dancing and drumming the evil spirits away, we must admit that compared with the methods of modern medicine the constant presence of the medicine man and his untiring ceremonial devotions for days and nights have a profound psychologic influence." Indian Service physicians were slow to recognize these benefits, although those entering the service in the 1940s better appreciated the values derived from medicinal herbs, massages, sweat baths and cathartics. Sweat baths and body massages used in some ceremonies also provided a physiotherapeutic benefit.[28]

Although there was an increased appreciation of traditional healers among some practitioners in the Indian health program, there were just as many—if not more—who were opposed to the healers and who remained skeptical of any traditional Indian healing practice. As a matter of official policy, Collier encouraged traditional Indian healing practices, even if medical personnel misunderstood them. When tribal customs were encouraged, the impersonal and rigid relations that were standard with hospital and clinical care decreased, minimizing the cultural gap between practioners and patients.[29]

Heightened cultural sensitivity was also an impetus for greater utilization of modern medicine by Indians. The physical location and aesthetics of new Indian Service facilities reflected this newfound sensitivity. During Collier's tenure, new hospitals were built facing east toward the rising sun, thereby incorporating an important cultural characteristic of many tribes. Other hospital facilities included small, rather than large, windows that were less revealing to outsiders who might peer into the facility.[30]

While there was greater acceptance of modern medicine, cultural barriers restricting utilization of hospitals and health services remained. Language challenges proved to be formidable. Although interpreters were widely used, they reduced much of the physician-patient interaction to impersonal comments. It was common for English words to lack adequate translations into the tribal language. In such circumstances, physicians were "unable to judge the patient's subtleties of expression, the tone of voice and inflection, the tone of a phrase which is so important in communicating emotional tone in English." These important verbal and non-verbal cues were lost in the stale translations allowed for in such settings.[31]

Facility Utilization

Commissioner Charles Burke once argued the critics of the Indian Service erroneously concluded the Indians were "not being properly cared for" and were "being neglected by the Government." In realty, the commissioner opined, it was the Indian who rejected or resisted change and, therefore, he was responsible for Congressional parsimony. Following this line of thinking, Burke may well have said Congress would not fund a program the Indians would not use anyway. While there was an element of truth in Burke's reasoning, he failed to consider the Indian Service's responsibility to educate the Indians regarding Western concepts of medicine. The commissioner was among those Lewis Meriam wrote about, in 1928, when he argued the government assumed some sort of magical education would occur once the Indians became landowners via land severalty. Burke clearly adopted a one-size-fits-all philosophy and expected the Indians to adapt their thinking and beliefs to it.

To his credit, Collier did more than any other commissioner of Indian affairs prior to 1960 to meld Western and Indian ways. The result was more tribal health boards initiated what would one day become known as community-based health care. With increased cultural sensitivity and wider acceptance of traditional Indian medicine, hospital and clinic utilization rates among Indians increased. Although not all Indians availed themselves of medical care, more Indians (proportionally) made use of hospitals and clinics than did the general population. In 1940, for example, 80% of all Indian babies were born in Indian Service operated or contracted hospitals. At the same time just 10% of comparable non-Indian economic groups made use of hospitals for childbirth, with only half of all women nationally entering a hospital for such care. Furthermore, one out of five Indians availed themselves of hospital care while just one of fifteen in the general population did.[32]

With the demand for expanded medical facilities, the American College of Surgeons began accrediting medical facilities nationwide. By 1942, twelve Indian Service hospitals were among the 2,261 hospitals approved across the country (out of 6,291 registered hospitals). Of those in Indian Country, seven were in Oklahoma and two were in New Mexico. This was a far cry over 1930 when no Indian Service facility met the criteria. Gaining accreditation was a challenge for Indian hospitals because of inadequate clerical assistance (record-keeping) and retaining "adequate and competent hospital personnel." Most Indian facilities were "inaccessible to cities and towns" and located in isolated areas, such as Alaska, the Southwest and the Northern Plains. Not surprisingly, Collier argued many physicians and nurses worked "under frontier conditions" that were far from ideal.[33]

By midcentury, forty-eight Indian Service hospitals housed an average of

1,746 patients per day, while the annual total of American Indians treated on an outpatient basis surpassed 418,000. Sixteen contract hospitals housed an average of 936 patients per day. Combined, contract and non-contract hospitals provided outpatient care to over 9,600 American Indians. Table 14 shows the health facilities available to American Indians in 1954.

Table 14

Health Facilities for American Indians: 1954

Contract Hospitals	Non-contract Hospitals	Indian Service Hospitals	Health Centers	Health Stations	Field Locations	School Infirmaries
16	12	48	18	62	148	13

(Source: *Health Services for American Indians*, 1957)

Increased utilization nearly overwhelmed Indian Service facilities, straining the overall effectiveness of the Division of Indian Health. In 1929, Assistant Commissioner Edgar Meritt requested twenty-five additional hospitals and fifty more "good doctors." Collier complained in 1944 that the program still had only 40% of the physicians necessary to provide basic care for American Indians and Alaska Natives. There remained an urgent need for public health nurses, particularly after World War Two, when one in seven positions were vacant. Staff shortages resulted in five hospitals being closed, in 1942-1943. Two additional hospitals had their capacity reduced as a matter of economy. Between 1940 and 1952, the Indian Service closed twenty-nine Indian hospitals, most of them outdated and obsolete.[34]

The increased utilization of hospitals and clinics did not in-and-of themselves improve health status. The growing number of services provided by the Public Health Service and other health prevention programs via state and local governments were responsible for much of this improvement. The Indian Service continued to receive on loan from the Public Health Service physicians, dentists, nurses and sanitary engineers. These healthcare professionals designed and implemented programs to safeguard water supplies, ensure sanitary sewage disposal, protect dairy herds, control venereal disease and encourage general well-being. To alleviate shortages, staff and facilities from the National Institutes of Health were also made available to the Indian health program.

Increased health education was important in increasing the utilization of medical services among the Indians. Although part of its educational program since 1910, it was not until the 1920s, when the American Red Cross and the American Child Health Association provided assistance that the Indian Service developed health courses for use in Indian schools. As part of the Indian New Deal, a Supervisor of Health Education was appointed to implement the first dental hygiene program for use in Indian schools and communities. Continued cooperation with state and local health departments, private organizations and universities made noticeable improvements in Indian health conditions, something acting medical director Burnet M. Davis told the Association of Military Surgeons was imperative. Speaking in November 1952, Davis made clear the official Indian Service goal was "to stimulate and assist states and counties to develop adequate local health services and to extend them to the reservation areas." [35]

Sanitation Deficiencies

Prior to 1940, sanitation efforts in Indian Country extended no further than occasional clean-ups, even though the Public Health Service Sanitary Engineering Corps provided assistance in surveying water and sewer systems for Indian Service hospitals and schools. Outside of these activities, little was done for individual American Indians and Alaska Natives, making sanitation the most neglected element of the Indian health program. In 1936, James Townsend lamented the lack of sanitation services. "There is no regular program of sanitation in the Indian health service," he opined, even though the "great need for sanitation exists among the smaller Indian villages, (which) usually obtain water in a nearby stream, spring or well which may be open to contamination." Most Indians had "no method of excreta disposal and those that do almost invariably use a privy of the surface type." In Alaska, the sanitary conditions were abominable. "Garbage and refuse disposal," Thomas Parron wrote in 1954, "generally is very primitive, consisting usually of dumping upon the ground surface or over river embankments." The existence of permafrost compounded refuse disposal. [36]

The fear of disease spreading beyond Indian Country was very real. In Nebraska, officials warned that health conditions among the Winnebago and Omaha Tribes were serious and, unless measures were undertaken to control disease, "the situation will seriously menace the whole county, if not the state." Due to such fears, Congress authorized the states to enforce their sanitation and quarantine laws on Indian lands beginning in 1929. The Secretary of the Interior granted state officials access to reservations to inspect health and sanitation conditions and enforce state quarantine regulations as provided by state law. In 1936, Franklin Roosevelt signed Executive Order no. 7369 granting legal sanction for deputizing Indian Service physicians as state health officers, leading many states to appoint government physicians to serve as deputy state health officers with the authority to enforce state health regulations on the reservations. Such authority served an additional function by encouraging states to assume a greater role in Indian health care. [37]

When Fred Foard was detailed by the Public Health Service to oversee the Division of Indian Health in 1948, he viewed the lack of basic sanitation as the single greatest culprit in the campaign to eliminate health hazards in Indian Country. At the time, there were only two sanitary engineers in Indian Country, and only one dedicated his full attention to public health work—and he was assigned exclusively to the Navajo Nation. To overcome these deficiencies, Foard relied on the assistance of the Public Health Service, which detailed H. Norman Old to the Division of Indian Health to serve as its first full-time environmental sanitary engineer. With the Indian Service, Old conducted forty-five environmental surveys in eighteen states and developed a framework for a service-wide sanitation program. In the process, he concluded the high mortality and morbidity rates among the Indians and Alaska Natives were the result of faulty sanitation. Diseases such as dysentery, diarrhea and enteritis were prevalent among infants and children, with protozoa infestations common.[38]

Old's surveys convinced the Indian Service of what appeared to be the obvious: Sanitation services among the Indians would have to take into account home and community conditions rather than focusing strictly on services at public facilities, such as schools. Among the challenges uncovered by Old were contaminated water supplies, improper excreta disposal, poor food sanitation and storage, vector and rodent problems and over-crowded homes. To overcome these challenges, Foard implemented a pilot training program in 1949 to encourage Navajo and Hopi men to serve as sanitary aides. Three years later, the Indian Service began training twelve Indian men for these positions. Under the direction of Hugh Eagan, the Public Health Service provided an eight-week in-service in Phoenix, Arizona, where the men were certified as aides. They then returned to their reservations where they began the task of demonstrating practical measures to raise the level of sanitation in Indian homes and communities. Within five years, seventy-five men were trained as sanitarian aides, with some receiving additional training from the Centers for Disease Control in Atlanta, Georgia.[39]

Inadequate sanitation facilities and the Indians' general lack of understanding contagion was no abstraction. Nowhere was this lack of comprehension more disturbing than in the Indian and Alaska Native morbidity and mortality rates. Diseases such as trachoma, tuberculosis, influenza, gastroenteric disorders, meningitis and others resulted from or were compounded by, unsanitary conditions. Improper excreta disposal and other human waste contributed to the spread of micro-organisms that precipitated outbreaks of dysentery, hepatitis and illnesses such as intestinal protozoa. Nothing less than a full-scale assault on environmental and sanitation deficiencies was needed.[40]

The Alaska Native Health Study

Overall conditions among Alaska Natives lagged far behind the Indians in the continental United States. A scarcity of elderly natives and a tuberculosis rate ten times greater than that of the territory, pointed to extreme health conditions. In 1953, in an attempt to gain an accurate picture of health within the native villages, the Alaska Territorial legislature and the Territorial Governor requested Thomas Parron of the University of Pittsburgh School of Public Health to make a thorough canvas of Alaska Native and non-native health conditions. In his study simply entitled "Alaska's Health: A Survey Report," Parron observed that Alaska was divided into two worlds: White Alaska and Native Alaska. While the health of white Alaskans paralleled that of the general population in the continental United States, the health of Alaska Natives was "deplorable and resemble[d] in some degree the conditions found in the United States at the turn of the [twentieth] century." Parron noted the Alaska Native Service, an extension of the Indian Service, traditionally, but unwisely, "confined its health program largely to curative and restorative services" rather than preventive services. The result was 90% of all tuberculosis deaths in the territory were Alaska Natives and 10% of all native infants died during their first year of life. [41]

To remedy the crisis, Parron recommended subdividing Native Alaska into six health service districts, five of which would be centered around the Alaska Native Service hospitals located at Point Barrow, Kotzebue, Bethel, Kanakanak and Tanana; the sixth would be serviced by a hospital in Nome. Each district was given maximum discretion in decision-making so as to be self-contained and provide the widest degree of administrative autonomy consistent with overall program and fiscal policy. [42]

An all-out campaign against tuberculosis using the new anti-tuberculosis drug isoniazid and BCG vaccinations and a commitment to tackle other health problems was initiated even before Parron released his report in 1954. But change and results came slowly and then mostly for those living near centers of population where services were more readily available. It was too common, Parron explained, for physicians to provide services with few supplies and a limited arrangement of surgical instruments. A complete renovation of Alaska Native health services was essential. Until then, health conditions among Alaska Natives would remain inferior to non-Indians and below those of American Indians. [43]

Need for a Paradigm Shift

As midcentury drew neigh, the health services available and care provided for American Indians and Alaska Natives remained woefully inadequate. What was necessary to elevate health conditions and care to an adequate level was a new paradigm, one that focused on an Indian Country-wide approach rather than sporadic, emergency-based services. Such an undertaking required, among others, a medical statistical service to tabulate, correlate and analyze morbidity, mortality and other vital statistics. This would encourage clinical research into specific pathogens and challenges facing Indian Country. Statistics and other medical data for outlining program goals and for determining methods to attain such goals were essential. The lone Indian Service statistician, J. Nixon Hadley, admitted data on health conditions were "remarkable for their paucity." The maintenance of a minimal level of health care was hampered by lack of data on base population (including age-sex data) and specific causes of morbidity and mortality. A medical statistical service was a constituent part of the overall paradigm shift required by the circumstances.[44]

By the early 1950s, the Division of Indian Health—while showing improvement over its pre-depression services—was ripe for integration with the Public Health Service. Congress was increasingly committed to terminating the federal-Indian relationship and eliminating Indian-specific programs. Beyond political considerations, a practical approach to improve Indian health care was to provide the responsibility to the Public Health Service, where expertise and funding was adequate. When Dillon Myer assumed the Indian commissionership in 1951, he unequivocally made known his intention to transfer the functions of the Indian Service "to the Indians themselves or to appropriate agencies of local, State or Federal Government." The era of termination began.[45]

Notes

1. Gessner, 218.

2. Between 1941 and 1945, a number of federal agencies were relocated from Washington, DC, to accommodate wartime industries. The Indian Service was reestablished in Chicago, diminishing its political influence. Prucha, *The Great White Father*, Vol. II, 1068-1069.

3. *Indian Health: A Problem and a Challenge* (Washington, DC: GPO, Branch of Health, Bureau of Indian Affairs), 1955. *Annual Report*, 1950, 343. Braasch, 221. HR 2860, May 11, 1929.

4. Gessner, 200-202.

5. *Hearings Before the Senate Committee on Indian Affairs on the Conditions of the Indians in the United States*, part 5, 1962, 2013, 2119.

6. *Hearings Before the Senate Committee on Indian Affairs on the Conditions of the Indians in the United States*, part 2, 554-555.

7. Meriam, 239.

8. Gessner, 245. Braasch, 222. H. Norman Old, "Sanitation Problems of the American Indians," *The American Journal of Public Health* (43, February 1953).

9. Braasch, 224-225, argued these social and economic indices increased in importance in those areas where "integration of the Indian with his white neighbor is possible." The American Medical Association strongly encouraged integration of the Indian into mainstream America.

10. H. DeLien and J. Nixon Hadley, "How to Recognize an Indian Health Problem," *Human Organization* (11:3, Fall 1952), 29-33. Maintaining accurate statistics was a concern that plagued the Indian medical service, one that lent credence to the transfer into the Public Health Service. Emerson, "Indian Health-Victim of Neglect," 219. *Annual Report,* 1937, 237. *Annual Report*, 1940, 383.

11. The focus on children was especially true in the fields of education and health care. Education and health were so closely intertwined that to do one was to do the other. Much of federal Indian policy affected adults (allotment, law and order, citizenship, economic development) but children were always the focal point. *Annual Report*, 1934, 95. In 1949, Moorman, 374, estimated there were 500 crippled Navajo children alone. He encouraged the Indian Service to hire orthopedic surgeons. "An Act to provide for the general welfare by establishing a system of Federal old-age benefits, and by enabling the several States to make more adequate provision for aged persons, blind persons, dependent and crippled children, maternal and child welfare, public health, and the administration of their unemployment compensation laws, to establish a Social Security Board; to raise revenue; and for other purposes," 49 Stat. 631, Title V, Part 2 "Services for Crippled Children." Section 511 defined the purpose and the conditions of coverage while section 515 provided for qualifications of state plans for federal assistance—plans that could be denied and left unfunded if not according to federal mandate. *Health Services for American Indians*, 163. In 1949, Arizona and New Mexico relented and provided such services, but only after an Arizona Supreme Court ruling determined that Arizona Indians were indeed state citizens entitled to vote. By implication, Arizona could no longer deny such services to its Indian citizens. *Harrison et al. v. Laveen*, (196 *Pacific Reporter* 456), July 15, 1948.

12. *Health Services for American Indians*, 165.

13. Foard, "The Health of the American Indians," 1404-1405. The American Medical Association recommended adequate numbers of pediatricians for Indian reservations. Moorman, 374.

14. *Annual Report*, 1954, 35.

15. Meriam, 558. Braasch, 223-225. Many mid-western Indian children consumed "great quantities of berries." This was especially true during the summer months. Despite warnings, the seasonal berry gorges continued—and resulted in intestinal complaints.

16. *Annual Report*, 1941, 434.

17. *Hearings Before the Senate Committee on Indian Affairs on the Conditions of the Indians in the United States*, Part 4, 1585-1589. Gessner, 228-229.

18. *Annual Report of the Secretary of the Interior*, 1943, 281. *Health Services for American Indians*, 178.

19. "Rehabilitation of the Navajo and Hopi Indians," *Hearings Before a Subcommittee of the Committee on Interior and Insular Affairs in the United States Senate* (Washington, DC: GPO, 1949), April 20, 1949, 94. Moorman, 371.

20. *Observations on Indian Health Problems and Facilities*, 35.

21. *Annual Report*, 1938, 241. Congress appropriated the funds with the understanding that the Navajo Tribal Council would reimburse the cost through tribal funds.

22. 64 stat. 826. This was particularly true after the Indian Health Transfer Act, although prior to the transfer the Public Health Service detailed more than fifty

commissioned corps officers (physicians and dentists) to the Indian Service.

23. Raup, 12. *Health Services for American Indians*, 154.

24. Raup, 157.

25. *Annual Report*, 1944, 249. McKay, "Rosebud Sioux Organize for Health."

26. Moorman, "Health of the Navajo-Hopi Indians." Adair, et al., "Patterns of Health and Disease Among the Navahos."

27. *Annual Report*, 1940, 380.

28. Leland C. Wyman and Flora L. Bailey, "Two Examples of Navaho Physiotherapy," *American Anthropologist* (46:3, 1944), 329-337. Moorman, 371-372.

29. John Adair and Kurt Deuschle, "Some Problems of the Physicians on the Navajo Reservation," Human Organization (16:4, Winter 1958), 21.

30. Urban Associates, Inc., *A Study of the Indian Health Service and Tribal Involvement in Health* (Washington, DC: GPO, Department of Health, Education and Welfare, 1974), 159.

31. Adair, et al., "Some Problems of the Physicians on the Navajo Reservation," 20.

32. "The Indian Service Health Activities," 6. *Annual Report*, 1941, 431.

33. "Indian Hospitals Ranked Among Nation's Best," 13-14. The most difficult criteria for Indian Service hospitals to meet were for chemical and bacteriological examinations, a serological and pathological service and an x-ray department. "Indian Service Hospitals Gradually Meeting Standards for Acceptance by the American College of Surgeons," 11-12. Post mortem examinations were difficult for Indians to accept since many were prejudiced against opening bodies after death for examination.

34. In 1944, there were 100 vacancies in the physician corps and 188 in the nursing corps. "Health Program of Indian Service," 32. Burnet M. Davis, "The Health Program of the Bureau of Indian Affairs," *The Military Surgeon* (112:3, March 1953), 73. Davis, who served as acting director of the Indian health program between October 1952 and July 1953, noted the Indian Service was utilizing non-government hospitals and private physicians for the care of Indians.

35. Davis, 172. Contracts with private and university radio stations sent health related messages over the air-waves to some isolated and scattered reservations across the West. Programs were also initiated for the first time for off-reservation Indian agricultural workers, emphasizing the control of tuberculosis, basic sanitation maintenance and healthy living environments.

36. Townsend, *Observations on Indian Health Facilities and Problems*, 31, 41. Parron, VI-29.

37. 45 stat., 1185. Executive Order 7369, May 13, 1936, *Federal Register*, Vol. 1, 405.

38. Foard, "The Health of the American Indians," 1404. *Annual Report*, 1952, 397. William B. Owens, Ralph F. Honess and James R. Simon, "Protozoal Infestations of American Indian Children," *Journal of the American Medical Association* (102:12, March 24, 1934), 913-915. Of the eighty-three Arapaho boys and seven adults tested, 93.7% were positive for intestinal protozoa. The presence of protozoa was blamed on poor housing, lack of plumbing fixtures and the practice of defecating in convenient but unsanitary places.

39. Old, 212.

40. Owens, et al.

41. Parron, III-1.

42. Parron, IV-32-34.

43. The Indian tuberculosis rate per 100,000 was 571.5. The overall national rate was 62.4. The Alaska Native rate was 2,452.4. *Indian Health Highlights* (Washington, DC: GPO, Public Health Service, 1964).

44. Foard, "The Health of the American Indians," 1405. "Rehabilitation of the Navajo and Hopi Indians," 97. DeLien and Hadley, 30, cite a number of case examples of where proper control groups were not established when conducting tests. In one such example, a large percentage of Indian school youth were classified as having syphilis, leading to cries of "moral indignation" by the press. Subsequent re-examinations showed the facts had not been properly determined and the public had been misinformed. This type of inadequate research only "created suspicion and distrust and was a definite disservice to the Indian." J. Nixon Hadley, "Health Conditions among Navaho Indians," *Public Health Reports* (70:9, September 1955), 831-836.

45. *Annual Report*, 1951, 353.

CHAPTER SEVEN

Into the Public Health Service

During the summer of 1953, a seasoned cardiologist and internal medicine specialist named James "Ray" Shaw became the director of the newly reorganized Branch of Indian Health. At the time Shaw was a twenty-year Public Health Service Commissioned Corps Officer who served as medical advisor on loan from the Public Health Service and as Director of the Division of Hospitals. As head of the Indian medical program, Shaw sought to integrate Indian health services with those of state and local governments. His foremost goal was to improve American Indian and Alaska Native health status, no small task for a people challenged by a "backlog of disease and disability accumulated through generations of neglect."[1]

To meet this goal, Shaw and Surgeon General Leonard A. Scheele aggressively advocated a transfer into the Public Health Service where there were better prospects for increased funding for hospital construction and services. It was essential to modernize and expand medical facilities if Indians were to have a fair chance to compete in the American economy. An expanded public health program to control communicable diseases was needed in order to raise the average Indian age of death, which remained at thirty-six years (compared to sixty-one for non-Indians). As importantly, Shaw tired of Public Health Service officials being subordinate to Indian Service bureaucrats. To make progress, Foard and Shaw agreed, was it too much to expect that the Public Health Service staff delivering such care administer the health program?[2]

Rekindling the Transfer Idea

By 1950, nearly every state and national medical organization favored the consolidation of the Indian health program with the Public Health Service, noting the latter provided a variety of services for the former. The Senate Committee on Indian Affairs discussed repealing the Indian Reorganization Act, which Collier championed as the means of restoring the virtues of tribal nations. The committee also inquired whether it was advantageous for the Indian medical service to be "part of a relief and welfare function appertaining to local government?" By 1953, Congress answered its own inquiry by calling for the termination of all federal programs for American Indians and the creation of the Department of Health, Education and Welfare.[3]

The end of World War II sparked a wave of conservatism and nationalism in the United States, adding momentum to the transfer issue. Under President Truman's Fair Deal, the executive branch considered integration, consolidation and elimination of duplicative government programs. In 1948, Truman established a federal commission to find ways of reducing government waste. Known as the Commission on the Organization of the Executive Branch of the Government and chaired by former President Herbert Hoover, the commission concluded state and local health authorities must assume a greater responsibility for public health functions in Indian Country.[4]

The commission recommended Indian Service hospitals and physicians charge fees for services rendered to Indians. Furthermore, it encouraged greater use of contract physicians and utilization of off-reservation hospitals that would be operated by the federal government, but only until state or local health authorities could assume responsibility for such care. More directly, the commission counseled Indian Service hospitals be converted into community hospitals as quickly as possible, an idea Interior Secretary Oscar Chapman supported as cost-savings and service-improvement measures. By following this path, the "gradual liquidation of [Indian Service] hospitals and the absorption of Indian patients into other Federal or non-Federal systems" would be hastened.[5]

Beginning in 1951, the Indian Service adopted the policy of not operating any hospital or clinic when care was available from state and local health facilities or where Johnson-O'Malley contracts for medical services could be consummated. Commissioner of Indian Affairs Dillon Myer enforced a policy of operating facilities only when Indians could not receive care elsewhere or could not receive care without being segregated. In effecting this policy, Myer closed the Fort Berthold Indian Hospital in August of 1951, and proposed closing seven more hospitals in 1952. A year later, he negotiated a contract with the State of South Dakota providing for the transfer of public health and preventive services in Indian Country to that state.[6]

Acting on the advice of the Hoover Commission and the critical need for hospital services in rural America, both chambers of Congress considered bills calling for construction of joint-use facilities. In 1949, Congressman Harold Patten (D-AZ) introduced HR 3635 authorizing non-Indians to use Indian Service hospitals. While supporting the concept of integration, Chapman recommended several modifications, including protecting Indian priority to services. When Congress enacted Public Law 291 in 1952, it incorporated Chapman's basic concerns and granted statutory authority to the secretary to transfer any Indian hospital to state or local agencies. It also gave the secretary authority—if the health needs of the Indians were better served—to enter into contracts with federal, state or territorial governments or political subdivisions thereof "providing for the transfer by the Indian Bureau of Indian hospitals or other health facilities."[7]

Indians retained service priority over non-Indians in any hospital that was transferred to outside authorities. The admittance of non-Indian patients, while authorized, was allowed only in areas where there were an insufficient number of hospital beds or health facilities available to serve them. Access was permissible only if Indians did not utilize such services. With the Indian Service seeking to economize and Congress granting legislative authority to close Indian hospitals—as well as the advent of the Bureau's relocation policy that forced many Indians from the reservations to urban centers—Myer and his successor Glenn Emmons closed eight Indian hospitals between 1951 and 1955.[8]

Mindful of its ultimate desire to consolidate services, the Indian Service established a new office of Public Health Services within the Branch of Indian Health. A trained public health physician was to direct the activities of the office, which was designed to administer and develop programs aimed at terminating the federal government's Indian-only health care responsibilities. Among its duties, the new office developed a comprehensive medical-dental program that incorporated provisions focused on effective tuberculosis control, which by 1956 consumed 40% of the Indian health budget.[9]

The fundamental goal of the public health program was to improve available services to American Indians and Alaska Natives and find ways to transfer those services (and responsibilities) to state and local agencies. Paralleling this goal was the aim of developing direct services from local agencies. In areas where care was unavailable, the Indian Service provided it, but only until state or local agencies assumed responsibility. In California, Wisconsin and Minnesota, public health services were provided under Johnson-O'Malley contracts. With nearly half of the Indians living in areas where local health services were either underdeveloped or non-existent, the Indian Service had few options but to continue providing services.[10]

When Congress approved of House Concurrent Resolution 108 in August of 1953, it called for termination of federal supervision for Indians "at the earliest possible time" and the abolition of all government facilities "whose primary purpose was to serve any Indian tribe or individual" that had been rendered unnecessary by the termination of such tribe. With the passage of Public Law 83-280 that same month, Congress conferred jurisdiction on several states for criminal and civil offenses involving Indians.[11] Although not directly related to health care, Public Law 280 and House Concurrent Resolution 108 established a Congressional intent of terminating federal responsibility for Indians, a proposition already apparent in the divestiture of some Indian health responsibilities to state and local governments.

The goal of transferring the Branch of Indian Health to the Public Health Service was one step toward the Congressional objective of divesting the Indian Service of all responsibility for American Indians and Alaska Natives. The Hoover Commission, which concerned itself with identifying the means of assimilating medical services into state or local health agencies, was an important impetus for change. But it was not the only agency—public or private—to recommend such consolidation. The American Medical Association long-favored consolidation and officials within the Public Health Service were rumored to threaten the withdrawal of assistance unless given full control of the Indian medical service. Not all health professionals agreed. While W.F. Braasch has reservations with the merger— arguing the mission of the Public Health Service was not the "general practice of medicine" but preventive medicine—he supported it if the Public Health Service retained a separate Indian budget and state boards of health assumed responsibility for preventive health measures.[12]

American Indian involvement in World War Two played an important role in the evolving Indian policy of the mid-twentieth century. Thousands of American Indians served in the war, which transformed the United States into an economic and military powerhouse. But it also mistakenly convinced the federal government that American Indians desired and were prepared to have all federal services terminated. The Indian Service even prepared a number of optimistic reports on Indian progress prompting Congress to begin termination and the consolidation of services.

Congress enacted dozens of laws repealing and/or terminating federal legislation related to American Indians. In March of 1952, Congressman Walter Judd (R-MN) introduced HR 6908, which called for transferring Indian health responsibilities and services to the Public Health Service. The following January, Senator Edward Thye (R-MN) introduced Senate Bill 132, which also called for the transfer of health services. These bills represented the first consolidation proposals since 1936, when Medical Director James Townsend unsuccessfully encouraged Collier and Ickes to work towards such a goal.[13]

The Indian Health Transfer Act

When the Senate concluded its fifteen-year investigation of Indian affairs in 1943, the Committee on Indian Affairs expressed its support for transferring Indian hospitals to the Public Health Service. With Congress preoccupied with the war, it was not until March 1947 that a bill was introduced calling for the transfer. Interior Secretary Julius Krug opposed the bill on the grounds the challenges of Indian administration were so closely related that it was inadvisable to separate health services from other Indian services. The Bureau of the Budget and the Federal Security Administration also opposed the bill and it was never reported out of committee and died.[14]

In 1949, Dr. William P. Shepard of the Metropolitan Life Insurance Company, a former president of the National Tuberculosis Association and then-president of the American Public Health Association, initiated a sustained effort to bring about the transfer. Assisted by Dr. James E. Perkins, Managing Director of the National Tuberculosis Association, and Noble J. Swearington, Shepard obtained the valuable endorsements of almost every major health organization in the country. Combined, these organizations applied sustained pressure on Congress to authorize the transfer. The American Medical Association, the American Public Health Association, the Association of State and Territorial Health Officers, the Governor's Interstate Council on Indian Affairs, the National Tuberculosis Association and numerous state agencies all rallied behind the proposal. A number of Indian tribes, including the Minnesota Chippewa, and the National Congress of American Indians and the Association on American Indian Affairs also supported the efforts of Shepard. In 1953, the House of Representatives approved Resolution 303, which recommended the transfer.[15]

Support for the move was premised on the assumption that the transfer would mitigate the chronic shortages in the physician and nursing corps of the Indian Service. In supporting a transfer, a Senate subcommittee pointed out that there were sixty Indian hospitals staffed by just sixty-three Indian Service physicians. To fill the need, eighty Public Health Service physicians were detailed to the Branch of Indian Health. It was readily apparent the Indian Service could not overcome its long-standing chronic shortage of personnel and likely would not without a policy change. On the other hand, the Public Health Service was a career organization offering what the Indian Service could not: Professional growth, fewer and shorter details to isolated health centers, better benefits and increased pay. The former was also able to recruit physicians and nurses more effectively than the latter, simply because of its career status and accredited health centers and hospitals. The Public Health Service encouraged and provided for post-graduate health research opportunities and study.[16]

With such a transfer, the Public Health Service would assume direct medical supervision of the Indian health program and, thereby, eliminate the inevitable conflicts that arose when superintendents exercised administrative control over health matters. On the Navajo Nation, for instance, Shaw complained that funds secured by the Branch of Indian Health to help fight tuberculosis were instead spent by the agency superintendent for a warehouse and community center. A transfer would also enable the Public Health Service to function as a nation-wide unit in accordance with professional evaluations of health needs and services and provide the Indian health program with leadership that was in tune with the challenges facing Indian Service physicians.[17]

As a professional and career organization, the Public Health Service could expand university relationships that would aid the campaign against poor health in Indian Country. Research into—and development of—preventive medicines would be more effectively instituted in the Public Health Service since it was single-mindedly focused on health issues. On the other hand, the Indian Service never solely focused on health as it was also concerned with Indian resources, land, education and other trust responsibilities. For Congress, economy and the elimination of duplicative health services was the driving force, although there was also the belief that only the Public Health Service could improve Indian health services.[18]

By turning responsibility for health care over to existing federal, state and local agencies, the Congressional goal of terminating Indian-only services began. Since the Public Health Service administered grants-in-aid for public health work, it understood the capacity of state and local health agencies to provide services for American Indians and Alaska Natives. It was also in a position to know the availability of state health programs and the extent to which American Indians received services available to them as American citizens. As part of the new Department of Health, Education and Welfare, the Public Health Service had direct access to other federal agencies that provided care under grants for maternal and child health, public assistance and other health related services.[19]

Support was not unanimous, as the departments of Interior and Health, Education and Welfare opposed the transfer. While the House debated the bill in 1953, the Interior Department voiced its opposition. "The various service programs for Indians are so closely related," Assistant Secretary Orme Lewis wrote Congressman A.L. Miller (R-NB), "that it is deemed inadvisable to separate the administration of the health services from the administration of other services to Indians." The following year, Interior dropped its opposition to the transfer and threw its weight behind the measure after it conceded the Public Health Service could more readily attain health objectives than the Indian Service. In a letter to Senator Hugh Butler (R-NB), Chairman of the Committee on Interior and Insular Affairs, Lewis wrote of the department's changed view. "Such a transfer would place the program in a department where decisions having to do with health and welfare of people could be readily and expeditiously made without the time-consuming process of negotiation of such matters between separate departments with divergent primary responsibilities."[20]

The Department of Health, Education and Welfare continued to oppose the transfer. Secretary Oveta Culp Hobby in a letter to Butler argued there had been good progress in transferring Indian responsibilities to state and local governments. The transfer, Hobby opined, would "increase the difficulties of pursuing the policy of integrating the Indians." Hobby feared a new administrative structure would be created in the Public Health Service to deal with Indians as "separate and distinct," leading to confusion in an Indian policy advocating incorporation of the Indians into American society. "The transfer of responsibility in itself would not constitute the solution to the health problems of the Indians," Hobby argued. "These problems are difficult and deep seated, involving the geographic location, economic status, cultural and educational levels and lack of social and political integration of this special segment of the Nation's population." The Bureau of the Budget also opposed the transfer, believing the move to be inconsistent with the intent of Congress to "integrate medical care for Indians with local health services."[21]

Numerous tribal councils and leaders opposed consolidation, fearing the liquidation of all federal services provided to Indians under treaty or statutory obligations. Francis Pipestem, Chairman of the Otoe Tribal Council, exhibited opposition representative of tribal leaders: the transfer was terminating and undermining the government-to-government relationship between the United States and tribal nations. The law did not "define the Federal responsibility for providing services to the Indians," Pipestem argued, and did not "authorize the Public Health Service (to) enter into agreements with the various tribes." Indian opposition, Congressman Walter Judd noted, was justified as "so often in the past, whenever any change was made in the existing pattern of care for them, they lost something."[22]

Despite objections, the House Committee on Interior and Insular Affairs made clear its desire to transfer the Indian health program as part of the overall termination of all federal responsibility for Indians. The Public Health Service carried the Branch of Indian Health for many years, the Committee concluded. National policy now "called for turning over this responsibility to State or local agencies wherever feasible—all aiming at erasing the line of distinction between services for Indians and the non-Indian population." Health was to be the first step in the complete liquidation of the Indian Service. State health agencies and national health groups emphasized the desirability of a transfer for many years. Now was the time, Senator Thye argued, as it would "improve the health services for the Indian people" and coordinate public health programs that would "further the long-range objective of the integration of the Indian people."[23]

The Oklahoma Congressional delegation remained an obstacle for the transfer. At the time, Oklahoma tribes received a "very high percentage" of all funds appropriated for Indian health care, largely because the Oklahoma Congressional delegation exerted considerable political clout in the Interior and Insular affairs committee. With strong opposition from the Oklahoma, the bill could not be reported out of committee and called before the House for a vote. Judd, however, remained vigilant in his efforts to see the bill enacted. When he caught the Oklahoma delegation missing a committee meeting after a late night party, Judd mustered the bill out of committee and before the House for a vote.[24]

Congress approved the Indian Health Transfer Act on August 5, 1954, and with President Eisenhower's signature the bill became law, taking effect in July 1955. Public Law 83-568 authorized the transfer of "all functions, responsibilities, authorities, and duties . . . relating to the maintenance and operation of hospital and health facilities for Indians, and the conservation of the health of Indians . . . (to) the Surgeon General of the United States Public Health Service." Indian Commissioner Glenn Emmons called the transfer "the biggest reduction of program responsibilities in the history of the [Indian] Bureau." On July 1, 1955, fifty-six hospitals, thirteen school infirmaries and 970 buildings valued at nearly $40,000,000, as well as some 3,500 health employees shifted from the Indian Service to the Public Health Service. To mitigate Indian fears over the closure of additional Indian hospitals, Congress prohibited the Public Health Service from closing any Indian health facility prior to July 1, 1956, unless the consent of the governing council of the affected tribe was secured. Any existing contractual arrangements between the Indian Service and state and local health agencies remained in effect. [25]

With the passage of the Indian Health Transfer Act, Public Law 291, which authorized the Secretary of the Interior to enter into contracts providing for the transfer of specific Indian health facilities to state or local governments, was repealed. Section two of the Transfer Act granted this authority to the Secretary of Health, Education and Welfare but added a provision that Public Law 291 did not include: the re-assumption of the management and operation of any hospital or clinic that did not provide adequate care to the Indians.

Settling into the Public Health Service

The transfer of the Branch of Indian Health was not expected to produce an immediate fiscal economy. In fact, Public Health Service officials, including Shaw, warned Congress that the transfer would temporarily increase the cost of the program. Nonetheless, with the transfer, a new era in Indian health care commenced, bringing increased appropriations, better services, more qualified personnel and an improved level of health among American Indians and Alaska Natives. [26]

The Branch of Indian Health was renamed the Division of Indian Health and placed within the Bureau of Medical Services. The division included an Office of the Division Chief and six branches: Hospital and Medical Services; Nursing Services; Sanitation Services; Field Health Services; Dental Services; and Program Analysis. The Hospital and Medical Services Branch provided medical care through Public Health Service Indian hospitals and contract facilities, while the Field Health Services Branch developed and oversaw the public health program, as well as administered non-hospital field facilities. The nursing, dental, and sanitation service branches were responsible for programs in their respective fields. Program Analysis reviewed and evaluated health statistics and data for program operations. All management and fiscal services were centered in the Bureau of Medical

Services.[27]

The area office structure of the Division of Indian Health intentionally resembled that of the Indian Service rather than paralleling the regional Public Health Service offices. This decision was based on the fact that the regional offices of the latter were far removed from centers of Indian population, whereas the offices of the former better approximated the Indian constituency served by the program. The close interrelationship between the health and other programs for Indians required the Division of Indian Health to have access to Indian Service area offices. Consequently, there were six area and three subarea offices established.[28]

With the expiration of Indian Service jurisdiction on June 30, 1955, Secretary of Health, Education and Welfare Marion B. Folsom issued regulations defining Indian eligibility for health services. The new regulations generally paralleled the Indian Service practice of local discretion in determining eligibility. Services were "available, as medically indicated, to persons of Indian descent belonging to the Indian community served by the local facilities and program, and non-Indian wives of such persons." An individual was eligible for services if the community in which he lived regarded him as Indian. Evidence of Indianness included tribal membership or enrollment, living on tax-exempt land, ownership of restricted property, active participation in tribal affairs or "other relevant factors" that the Indian Service recognized as constituting membership. Doubtful cases were left to the discretion of the medical officer in charge of the facility. Individuals "clearly able to pay the cost of hospital care" were expected to do so, with some services being conditioned upon payment. No fees were charged for preventive services, such as immunization shots, health exams for school children and prenatal clinical visits.[29]

To obtain outside advice on the operation of the program, Surgeon General Scheele created an Advisory Committee on Indian Health in 1956. The nine member committee, which included three American Indians, evaluated the effectiveness of the Indian health program in light of cultural and welfare considerations. A second committee, the Interconstituent Committee on Services to Indians, was established that same year in an effort to coordinate the medical program with related federal, state and local programs serving American Indians and Alaska Natives. This committee concerned itself with the issue of eligibility for services and increasing Indian utilization of other available health services, both of which were important since the Public Health Service took the position that no Indian had a "legal entitlement to medical services."[30]

Health Services for American Indians and Alaska Natives

As head of the Division of Indian Health, Shaw and the Public Health Service needed additional fiscal resources if they were to successfully reduce ill health. They found an ally in Congress during the 1956 Indian health appropriation hearings. Believing the end of Indian-only services was at hand, Congress was willing to appropriate funds if the Public Health Service quantified the time needed to prepare the Indians for assimilation. The House Appropriations Committee explained Indians were provided health services for over a hundred years but were "still the victim of an appalling amount of sickness." Staff housing was lacking or inadequate and the workload of medical professionals was testing their "patience and endurance." This all pointed to "a gross lack of resources equal to the present load of sickness and accumulated neglect." The problem, the committee agreed, could not be approached with timidity. The full extent of the need, the time frame to correct the challenge and the costs involved had to be determined.[31]

The committee asked Folsom for a comprehensive evaluation of Indian health care and the resources to elevate Indian health conditions to an "acceptable" level. Congress was willing to appropriate funds but predicated such appropriations on the creation of baseline data. Time was of the essence, for if Indians were to be emancipated from federal supervision and services, they first had to be free of disease. Aided by the Indian Service and scholars from five universities, Folsom submitted the requisite reports to Congress in April of 1957. The final report was uncanny in its similarities to earlier health studies. "Indians of the United States today have health problems resembling in many respects those of the general population of the nation a generation ago." Diseases largely controlled among the nation-at-large still caused widespread illness and death among American Indians. Table 15 illustrates the ten most reported communicable diseases among American Indians and Alaska Natives at the time of the transfer.[32]

Table 15

Ten Most Reported Communicable Diseases: 1952-1954
(Per 100,000 Population)

Disease	Indians in Continental U.S.	Alaska Natives
Influenza and Pneumonia	2,906	2,957
Dysentery	857	N/A
Measles	842	4,850
Tuberculosis	643	2,094
Gonorrhea	467	1,267
Syphilis	385	116
Trachoma	279	557
Chicken pox	249	1,345
Mumps	213	1,579
Whooping Cough	128	N/A

(Source: *Public Health Service Survey*, 1957 and *Alaska Health Survey*, 1954)

The causes of the egregious health conditions were varied and included inadequate health services, substandard and overcrowded housing and a lack of adequate sanitation facilities. The health challenges with the greatest urgency were tuberculosis, pneumonia and other respiratory diseases, diarrhea and other enteric diseases, accidents, eye and ear diseases, dental disease and mental illness.[33] To bring the level of health to an acceptable standard, the Public Health Service announced a comprehensive preventive health program. Closely allied with this was the need to correct gross environmental sanitation deficiencies in Indian homes and communities, which was done through a federally supported construction program. Former director Fred Foard argued this in 1949, connecting typhoid, diphtheria, diarrhea and other diseases with poor sanitation. A sanitation program was to be the cornerstone of preventive health.[34]

The Public Health Service redefined sanitation deficiencies by placing them in five broad categories. A prime cause of disease was the lack of domestic water, which necessitated the transportation of water from distant communal sources. The continued use of contaminated water sources for domestic purposes compounded matters. Lack of insect vector control (resulting from improper waste and refuse disposal), unsafe excreta disposal (causing parasitic infections) and a general lack of basic sanitation practices within the home all decimated Indian communities. Overcrowded and poorly repaired houses, many of which still had earthen floors, hampered mitigation efforts. In 1950, Indian families remained four times as crowded as non-Indian families (2.2 Indians per room versus 0.6 non-Indians per room). Reservations were also dispersed in isolated areas. The Tohono O'odham in Arizona, for example, lived in seventy-three villages, half of which were inaccessible by graded roads. Except for the agency town of Sells and a few surrounding villages, none of the villages on the 2.8 million acre reservation had electricity, and domestic water was imported from as far as ten miles away.[35]

A preventive health program that included additional health facilities and a sanitation facilities construction project was essential to elevating Indian health conditions. Folsom estimated five to ten years' time to raise health status to an acceptable level. Thereafter, the federal health program could be progressively scaled back as the effects of the preventive and sanitation services and facilities lessened the impact of communicable diseases. This would allow state and local governments, as well as the Indians themselves, to assume responsibility for health services.[36]

The Public Health Service was mindful to couch the preventive program within the context of the overall health conditions of the Indians. In his report to Congress, Folsom stressed Indian health concerns were more than just an issue of health. "To achieve good health," the secretary wrote, "Indians need more than measures aimed directly at disease prevention and control. They need better general education, vocational training, housing, food, roads, and means of transportation." In addition to these physical needs, there were deep social and cultural issues to be considered. "They need more understanding and acceptance by the rest of the population, particularly their own non-Indian neighbors." If any one component of the delicate puzzle were ignored, the challenge would be prolonged. The annual costs of operating such a program would be $60 to $65 million, not including $45 million spread over a ten-year period to improve hospitals, clinics and housing. An additional $29 million was needed to construct sanitation facilities. [37]

The report convinced Congress of its fiduciary obligation to insure a minimal level of health care. More and better-qualified staff was hired and a wider array of services provided. Shaw focused his energies on constructing new hospitals and satellite facilities or contracting for such services. A wider battery of facilities was critical to improve the overall quality of health care if preventive health services were to take root as part of the broader community health services.

The Indian Health Facilities Act

Just two months after the report was issued to Congress, Senator Lee Metcalf (D-MT) and Congressman Leroy Anderson (D-MT) introduced two health facilities bills. Almost immediately, an amended bill prepared by the Public Health Service and reintroduced by Anderson replaced these bills. The modified bill authorized the Surgeon General—after consultation with tribal nations—to provide financial assistance to public or other non-profit organizations for the construction of community hospitals if such facilities provided services to Indians. The Public Health Service would provide local governments or non-profit groups planning to construct a hospital a sum of money equal to the proportion of the Indian population in the area. The Bureau of the Budget, which opposed the transfer, enthusiastically supported this bill, viewing it as "ultimately furnish[ing] health services to Indians in the same manner as they are provided to the rest of the population." [38]

Urged on by Foard, Metcalf and others, Congress enacted into law the Indian Health Facilities Act, in 1957. Known as Public Law 85-151, the act granted the Surgeon General statutory authority to use Indian health funds to construct joint-use community hospitals whenever he "determine[d], after consultation with Indians, that the provision of financial assistance to one or more public or other non-profit agencies or organizations for the construction of a community hospital constitutes a method of making needed hospital facilities available for such Indians which is more desirable and effective than direct Federal construction." [39]

The law had a dual purpose. Because of the age, condition, obsolescence and type of construction of many Indian health facilities inherited by the Public Health Service, the Surgeon General, in order to properly discharge his responsibilities, would have to immediately replace a dozen or more outdated and ill-repaired Indian hospitals. This was a political challenge of considerable magnitude given that Congress was no longer interested in funding Indian-only services. Moreover, providing adjacent non-Indian communities lacking financial resources with joint-use facilities fostered the Congressional objective of assimilating American Indians.[40]

Shaw enthusiastically supported the bill. Committed to integration of the Indians, Shaw recognized the remote location of most Indian reservations and their small population would mean "an extremely small hospital" if services were segregated. One-third of the Indian hospitals already had fewer than thirty beds, with another third having fewer than forty. "For hospitals of this size," Shaw argued, "it is not possible to provide staffs and ancillary services sufficient to meet the array of complicated medical problems inherent in the Indian health situation."[41]

The Indian Health Facilities Act did not authorize any new expenditures of funds but simply allowed Indian facility monies to be used for the construction of joint-use hospitals. By granting discretionary authority to the Surgeon General to undertake cooperative projects with non-Indian communities, the campaign against disease was intensified. Financial assistance was limited to the reasonable cost of the community facility attributed to Indian health needs, as determined by the Surgeon General. Community hospitals remained eligible for federal funding under the Hill-Burton Program, which made grants available for community health facilities. While constructed with federal funds, such hospitals were not under federal supervision, maintenance, administration or control, although signed agreements were required to guarantee they were open to American Indians.[42]

To insure his statutory charge of conserving the health of the Indians was carried out, the Surgeon General ordered Shaw to evaluate all health facilities available to American Indians and Alaska Natives and determine which areas could be served by community facilities rather than direct federal services. Shaw classified Indian hospitals into three categories: those acceptable and meeting state criteria for standards; those potentially acceptable and failing state criteria but having construction funds available to improve the facilities; and those not acceptable and not meeting state standards and having no funding available for repairs. Using this criteria, Shaw categorized twenty-four acceptable, thirteen potentially acceptable and seventeen not acceptable Indian hospitals. To forestall the closure or reduction of capacity in any hospital, the Public Health Service could not curtail any tuberculosis or pediatric services until the Indian tuberculosis and infant mortality rates were comparable with non-Indian rates.[43]

The intent of the study was to define an "orderly and timely development" of health facilities construction, something the Indian Service had never done. In so doing, Shaw established a priority list based on bed needs unmet and adjusted by several factors, including tribes considered nearest to having federal supervision withdrawn and their proximity to private and/or parochial health facilities. In the first seven years of Public Health Service administration, fourteen community hospitals and seven new or replacement Public Health Service Indian hospitals were constructed and four hospitals were modernized. The Gallup (New Mexico) Indian Hospital became the first designed to be a referral and consultation center for the greater Southwest.[44] Table 16 identifies the priority rank established by the Division of Indian Health and the number of beds needed and whether such beds could be provided via Indian Health Service hospitals, Community hospitals or undetermined hospitals.

Table 16

Priority List of Proposed Construction and Modernization of Hospitals, 1958

Service Unit	Rank	Number of Additional Beds needed in:		
		PHS	Community	Undetermined
Turtle Mountain	1	36		
Navajo	2	113		
San Carlos	3	36		
Standing Rock	4	27		
Fort Peck	5		25	
Red Lake	6			21
White Earth	7		16	
Mescalero	8			13
Jicarilla	9			12
Fond Du Lac	10		8	
Mole Lake	11		4	
Nett Lake	12		3	
Grand Portage	13		2	
Elko-Ruby Valley	14		4	
Hoopa Valley	15		15	
Colorado River	16		30	
Fort McDermitt	17		2	
Wind River	18		15	
Lac de Flambeau	19		4	
Fort Berthold	20		10	
Pima	21	28		
Fort Totten	22		5	
Papago	23			22
Mt. Edgecumbe	24		13	
Pine Ridge	25		8	
Anchorage	26		33	
Flathead	27		5	
Navajo	28	25		
TOTAL		265	202	68

(Source: Division of Indian Health, 1958)

The Indian Sanitation Facilities Construction Act

While the health survey stimulated a building program, it also pointed to a number of continuing health challenges, most notably sanitation services. It was a long-known fact in Indian Country that sanitation facilities were sorely lacking. In 1955, there were just thirteen sanitary engineers and sanitarians in the Indian health program assisted by thirty-one Indian sanitarian aides. No other resources were available to mitigate environmental deficiencies.[45]

Throughout the 1950s, sanitary engineers and Indian sanitarian aides conducted reservation-wide sanitation surveys. More than 80% of Indian and Alaska Native families hauled or otherwise imported domestic water supplies, with over 70% of this water coming from contaminated or likely contaminated sources. Less than 20% of Indian homes were equipped with adequate waste disposal, with 12% having no facilities at all. Post-neonatal infant mortality remained five times the non-Indian rate.[46]

While sanitation was essential for improving Indian health, the Surgeon General lacked authority to construct and maintain sanitation facilities for Indians. He was further hampered in that if he could construct such facilities (and he was legally impotent to do so) they would be built on Indian land under the jurisdiction of the Indian Service. Fragmented authority vested the Public Health Service with responsibility to conserve the health of the Indians without granting it authority to construct sewage and water supply facilities. To complicate matters, the Interior Department possessed the authority to construct sanitation facilities but was powerless to transfer such projects to state, local or tribal entities.[47]

To untangle the jurisdictional web, a series of meetings were held between officials of the Public Health Service, Department of Health, Education and Welfare, Indian Service, Department of the Interior, and the Office of Management and Budget. Out of these meetings came a concerted effort to secure the legislative authority for the Surgeon General to construct and maintain sanitation facilities. Included in the proposals was a proviso authorizing the Surgeon General to acquire non-Public Health Service land for use in such facilities. In January of 1956, Folsom held a meeting with select members of Congress to solicit bipartisan support for Indian sanitation facilities legislation. From this dialogue came the introduction of several bills in the 85th Congress for specific tribes. One of these bills became law in 1957, and authorized the Surgeon General to construct sanitation facilities for Elko Indian Colony in Nevada.[48]

The Elko legislation did not address the matter of authorizing the Surgeon General to construct and maintain sanitation facilities throughout Indian Country. Without such authorization, Congress had to enact legislation on a project-by-project basis. In April of 1958, acting Secretary of Health, Education and Welfare Elliot Richardson requested Congress prepare a bill granting the Surgeon General universal authority to construct such facilities in Indian Country. Although the bill died at the end of the 85th Congress, it was reintroduced along with eight other similar bills in 1959. Secretary of Health, Education and Welfare Arthur Fleming exhorted Congress to provide the Surgeon General with broad authority to construct sanitation facilities. "Few families and few communities," the secretary wrote Congressman Oren Harris (D-AR), "are able to . . . provide essential sanitation facilities from their own resources."[49]

On July 31, 1959, the Indian Sanitation Facilities Construction Act became law, providing the Surgeon General statutory authority to construct sanitation projects to mitigate "the serious environmental problems" in Indian Country. Public Law 86-121 amended the Indian Health Transfer Act by authorizing the Surgeon General to "construct, improve, extend, or otherwise provide and maintain, by contract or otherwise, essential sanitation facilities, drainage facilities, and sewage and waste disposal facilities . . . for Indian homes, communities, and lands." The Surgeon General was authorized to acquire land or rights-of-way for constructing sanitation facilities and, upon the completion of the facility, transferring it "to any State or Territory or subdivision or public authority thereof, or to any Indian tribe, group, band or community." Any domestic improvements were transferred to the occupant of the Indian home so served.[50]

The passage of the law would not in its own right relieve the environmental deficiencies among the Indians. "Sanitation improvements at reservation areas depend first upon acceptance by the Indians of modern concepts of the interrelationship between disease and insanitary living conditions," Fleming informed Harris, "and, second, upon provision and use of basic sanitation facilities—safe water supplies, safe sewage disposal and refuse disposal facilities." These tasks would not be easily accomplished among some tribes. A 1954 study in Arizona found assistance difficult to render because of deep-seated Indian "resistance to change." The same study concluded resistance occurred because of entrenched social attitudes and "habitual patterns of living" that were contrary to effective, modern preventive health measures. Recognizing individuals might accept change, the authors of the study argued community acceptance would be more difficult—and community acceptance was foundational for a sound preventive program to be successful.[51]

Signs of Progress

The operational improvements of the Division of Indian Health were significant during its first years in the Public Health Service. While there were challenges, initial signs pointed toward progress. Additional medical staff, including specialists from nearly every field of medicine, and improved and modernized health facilities made an impact. In the first years of Public Health Service responsibility, the full-time medical staff of the Indian health program grew 45%, passing the 5,000 mark. Physicians more than doubled to 300 and included pediatricians, surgeons and maternal and childhood specialists. The number of dentists tripled to 100, as did dental assistants and technicians. Sanitary Engineers and sanitarians increased from fourteen to sixty-eight, and sanitarian aides more than doubled to sixty-eight. Graduate nurses increased from 783 to 890, with practical nurses growing from 289 to 486. Pharmacists, medical social workers, community workers, medical records librarians, dietitians and nutritionists all increased four- or five-fold. The urgency and the need were so real that *espirit de corps* was at its peak. For the first time, it appeared the Division of Indian Health might provide comprehensive care to American Indians and Alaska Natives. [52]

In an effort to make health care more relevant, the Public Health Service expanded training opportunities for American Indians and Alaska Natives. Nurses trained at the School of Practical Nursing in Albuquerque, New Mexico, while advanced training was available at Shiprock, New Mexico, and Rapid City, South Dakota. Dental technicians received training at four facilities in the West and sanitarian aides were trained at Sandia Pueblo, New Mexico. Within five years, over one-half of the employees of the Indian health program were American Indian or Alaska Native, although most were in support staff roles, such as aides.

Table 17
Tuberculosis Incidence Rates: 1954-1959
(Per 100,000 population)

Year	Indian	Alaska Native	All People Groups
1954	571.5	2,452.4	62.4
1955	563.2	2,325.7	60.1
1956	474.3	2,283.8	54.1
1957	426.9	1,649.7	51.0
1958	421.8	978.7	47.5
1959	338.2	1,048.0	42.6

(Source: *Indian Health Highlights*, 1964)

The expansion of services, increasing appropriations, growing number of medical specialists and legislatively sanctioned construction projects meant nothing if Indian health conditions did not improve. In order to determine improvement of health conditions, the effectiveness of the program had to be measured. When viewed in this light, the Public Health Service made important advances in reducing the incidence of tuberculosis and infant mortality rates. Overall, Indian health conditions remained a generation behind the national standard, with Alaska

Native health conditions lagging by two generations. Diseases controlled among non-Indians were still the cause of disproportionate numbers of American Indian and Alaska Native deaths.

The most dramatic reduction in Indian Country was the incidence rate from the old Indian nemesis tuberculosis, which declined 49% among American Indians (571.5 to 292.3 per 100,000) and 78% among Alaska Natives (2452.4 to 547.5 per 100,000) with the introduction of antibiotics and improved health education. Although it was the leading cause of death among American Indians and Alaska Natives in 1949, the tuberculosis mortality rate declined so sharply that by the late 1950s it dropped to the ninth leading cause of death.[53] Table 17 shows the declining incidence rate of tuberculosis.

Corresponding with the decreasing tuberculosis rate was a declining infant mortality rate, which was aided by more hospital deliveries. Between 1954 and 1962, the mortality rate for Indian infants declined 36%, yet remained one and a half times higher than the non-Indian rate. Among Alaska Natives the infant death rate was double the Indian rate and triple the overall national rate. For post-neonatal infants the rate was even higher. The Indian rate of twenty-six deaths per 1,000 live babies was nearly four times the overall rate of seven deaths. The leading causes of infant mortality remained respiratory, digestive, infective and parasitic diseases.[54]

Owing to some improvement in sanitation matters, progress was also made in reducing gastroenteric diseases. Although the death rate from such diseases diminished among American Indians, it doubled among Alaska Natives. With non-Indians six times less likely than American Indians and Alaska Natives to experience such challenges, it was apparent that gastroenteric diseases remained a major contributor to ill-health among the Indians. Biliary disease was also significantly higher among American Indians than non-Indians.[55]

By 1959, the leading causes of death were new to Indian Country. Heart disease, accidents, influenza, pneumonia, gastroenteric diseases, malignant neoplasms, cirrhosis of the liver, vascular lesions of the central nervous system, as well as chronic diseases such tuberculosis were double or more the non-Indian rates. American Indians and Alaska Natives were less likely than non-Indians to be afflicted with malignant neoplasms, heart disease and vascular lesions, largely because they did not live as long and consequently did not face many of these geriatric diseases. Nonetheless, rates for these diseases were increasing. Table 18 compares the mortality rates of the five leading causes of death among American Indians and Alaska Natives with those of non-Indians.

The reduction in morbidity and mortality from several diseases, particularly tuberculosis, was reflected in an increased average life span among American Indians. Between 1954 and 1962 the average age at death for Indians rose from thirty-eight to forty-three, but among Alaska Natives it remained at just thirty years of age. With more services and better care, life expectancy among

American Indians also increased, rising from fifty-one to sixty-two. American Indian life expectancy, however, was still short of the non-Indian life expectancy of seventy years of age.[56]

Table 18

Top Five Causes of Death among American Indians and Alaska Natives:
1956-1960
(Per 100,000 Population)

| Disease | Rates for American Indians/Alaska Natives | | U.S. All | |
	1956-58	1958-60	1959	1960
Accidents				
U.S.	154.1	151.1	52.2	52.3
Alaska	183.0	181.5	115.2	110.5
Heart Disease				
U.S.	139.3	142.7	363.4	369.0
Alaska	95.4	77.1	111.5	118.1
Influenza/Pneumonia				
U.S.	93.8	82.8	31.2	37.3
Alaska	130.1	117.3	39.8	44.2
Malignant Neoplasms				
U.S.	63.7	67.1	147.4	149.2
Alaska	58.1	57.0	57.1	52.2
Infant Disease*				
U.S.	57.0	50.2	26.2	25.8
Alaska	N/A	74.0	42.9	40.5

*Per 1,000 Live Births
**Less than ten total deaths
(Source: *Indian Health Highlights*, 1964)

While health care improved, Indian health indices remained far behind those of non-Indians. Tuberculosis, gastroenteric and infant mortality rates all declined, although morbidity rates for these and other diseases remained high. The geographical isolation, social and linguistic barriers, cultural differences, environmental or sanitary hazards, lack of economic resources and the proclivity of American Indians and Alaska Natives to accept Western medicine still affected the overall health of the people and complicated the implementation of a comprehensive community health program. Added to these challenges were transportation difficulties, both for Indian patients and medical personnel, and the continued overlay of an imposed health care system that did not always consider the cultural views and needs of its clients.[57]

While there was progress in the formative years of Public Health Service responsibility, additional progress was dependent upon the increasing utilization of, and appropriations for, sanitation facilities and improved preventive health measures. While *espirit de corps* was high, it yet remained to be seen if the Public Health Service would do a better job of melding traditional Indian medicine and practices with Western ways.

Notes

1. Shaw succeeded Fred Foard, who retired from the Public Health Service in October 1952 to become director of the North Carolina State Department of Health. "Medical News" *Journal of the American Medical Association* (150:16) December 20, 1952, 1614. Shaw assumed command of the Branch of Indian Health on July 31, 1953 and was assisted by Dr. Frank French and Dr. Joseph Dean. "Government Services" *Journal of the American Medical Association* (152:14) August 1, 1953, 1357. *Annual Report of the Secretary of Health, Education and Welfare*, 1960, 132.

2. "Washington News," *Journal of the American Medical Association* (158:11), July 16, 1955, 14. Fred T. Foard, "The Federal Government and American Indians' Health," *Journal of the American Medical Association* (142:5), February 4, 1950, 328.

3. "The Indians' Health and Public Health," *American Journal of Public Health* (44:11), November 1954, 1461-1463. The Journal saw obvious advantages in placing the health program under the "immediate and sole direction" of Public Health Service professionals. Advantages included obtaining new facilities, equipment and technology; unshared control of funds by medical officers who understood better than the Indian Service bureaucrats the needs of a public health program; easier access to all the special skills and the broad competencies of the Public Health Service; and staffing benefits. Hazards could include the Public Health Service competing with itself for medical funds, both in terms of allocation and authorizations. "Aspects of Indian Policy," Senate Committee on Indian Affairs, Senate Committee Print, 79th Congress, 1st session (Washington, DC: GPO, 1945), 4, 16.

4. Fixico, 49. The Hoover Commission recommended a new Department of Natural Resources for all remaining Indian programs. Indian affairs would be part of this department, which would primarily emphasize national conservation and development of forests, water and other natural resources.

5. Authority already existed in the 1938 legislation that provided for the collection of fees from those Indians able to pay. 52 stat. 311. "Providing For Medical Services to Non-Indians in Indian Hospitals," *House Report no. 641*, 82nd Congress, 1st session, June 25, 1951, 2-3. Chapman argued such a law would help recruit physicians because they would provide care to a "greater variety of patients" and would be able to increase their pay

through private practice on the side (while still being contractually bound to provide care for Indians). An initial bill passed the House on June 20, 1949, but the Senate failed to take action. *Commission on the Organization of the Executive Branch of Government: Functions and Activities of the National Government in the Field of Welfare* (Washington, DC: GPO, 1949), 66. The Hoover Commission suggested detailing Public Health Service physicians to the Indian Service for a minimum of three and preferably four or five years so they would better understand the needs of the Indian community they served.

6. *Annual Report of the Secretary of the Interior*, 1952, 395. Myer argued final decisions regarding the closing of any health facility would not be made without tribal consultation. Nine community or sectarian hospitals provided care at Fort Berthold, with a small agency health staff maintained for residual needs. The tribal council, State health council, the State hospital, medical and pharmaceutical associations and the State Commission on Indian Affairs all approved the plan. *Annual Report of the Secretary of the Interior*, 1953, 34. New contracts were also signed expanding state and county services to Indians.

7. "Providing for Medical Services to Non-Indians in Indian Hospitals and for other Purposes," *House Report no. 797*, 81st Congress, 1st session, June 14, 1949. The revised bill (HR 4815) allowed physicians to contract for services but without becoming federal employees, prioritized Indian access to services and provided procedures for the disposition of funds from non-Indian patients. "Providing for Medical Services for Non-Indians in Indian Hospitals," *Senate Report no. 1095*, 81st Congress, 1st session, September 20, 1949. 66 stat. 34.

8. The closing of hospitals was not without anxiety. The fact remained that when hospitals closed, Indians lost their traditional services and had to apply to county or state health departments for medical attention. Many Indians, especially in Oklahoma, feared discrimination and the red tape involved and threatened to go it alone. Fixico, 46. Public Law 291 (HR 1043) was reported (2229), passed the Senate (2747), examined and signed (2869 and 2873), sent to the President (3091) and approved (3756) in the *Congressional Record* (98), 1952.

9. "Urgent Deficiency Appropriation Bill, 1956," *Hearing before the Committee on Appropriations, United States Senate on HR 9063*, 84th Congress, 2d session, March 16, 1956, 480.

10. *Annual Report of the Secretary of the Interior*, 1953, 36.

11. "Concurrent Resolutions: Indians," 67 stat. B132 (1953). "An Act to confer jurisdiction on the States of California, Minnesota, Nebraska, Oregon and Wisconsin, with respect to criminal offenses and civil causes of action committed or arising on Indian Reservations within such states, and for other purposes," 67 stat. 588.

12. Braasch, 221.

13. *Congressional Record* (98), 1952, 1900. Representative Harold A. Patten (D-AZ) also introduced legislation (HR 7232) to effect the transfer.

14. "Survey of Conditions among the Indians of the United States," *Senate Report no. 310: Analysis of the Statement of the Commissioner of Indian Affairs in Justification of Appropriations for 1944, and the Liquidation of the Indian Bureau* 78th Congress, 1st session, June 11, 1948, 9, 22. "Transfer the Maintenance and Operation of Hospitals and Health Facilities for Indians to the Public Health Service," *Senate Report no. 1530*, 83rd

Congress, 2d session, June 8, 1954, 9. Subcommittee hearings were held on March 28, 1948. The Bureau of the Budget, which surveyed the Indian health program in 1948, expressed the need for a new approach to Indian health problems but did not favor the transfer (16).

15. James R. Shaw, "Indian Health in Historical Perspective," unpublished paper courtesy of the author, University of Arizona, Tucson, October 18, 1982, 12. "Committee on Legislation," *Journal of the American Medical Association* (152:2), May 9, 1953, 169; (149:3), May 17, 1952, 283; (151:9), February 28, 1953; and (155:8), June 19, 1954, 753. *Transfer of Indian Hospitals and Health Facilities to Public Health Service, Hearings Before a Subcommittee of the Committee on Interior and Insular Affairs United States Senate on HR 303*, 83rd Congress, 2nd session, 1954.

16. "Organizational News," *Journal of the American Medical Association* (149:3), May 17, 1952, 283. "Transfer the Maintenance and Operation of Hospitals and Health Facilities for Indians to the Public Health Service," *House Report no. 870*, 83rd Congress, 1st session, July 17, 1953, 3-4.

17. John Todd, Interview with Dr. James R. Shaw, Unpublished Document in the Commissioned Corps Centennial Archives, History of Medicine Division, Library of Medicine, Bethesda, Maryland, 1988.

18. *Senate Report no. 1530*, 8. Shortly after the transfer, the Public Health Service announced it had contracted with the Phipps Institute of the University of Pennsylvania for a three-year health project designed to reduce tuberculosis among the Jicarilla Apache, Consolidated Utes, United Pueblo Tribes and the Mescalero Apache. "Government Services: Public Health Service," *Journal of the American Medical Association* (160:7), February 18, 1956, 576.

19. *Senate Report no. 1530*, 8. Both the Consolidated Ute Tribe and the Southern Ute Tribe contracted with Blue Cross-Blue Shield for their health care needs in 1955. "Urgent Deficiency Appropriation Bill 1956," 464. Raup, 26.

20. Orme Lewis to A.L. Miller, May 5, 1953, in *House Report no. 870*. Lewis to Hugh Butler, May 27, 1954, *Senate Report no. 1530*, 10.

21. Oveta Culp Hobby to Hugh Butler, May 28, 1954, *Senate Report no. 1530*, 17. "Hearings on the Proposed Transfer of Indian Hospitals and Health Facilities to the Public Health Service," *Hearings before the Committee on Interior and Insular Affairs United States Senate*, 83rd Congress, 2d session, May 28 & 29, 1954, 9.

22. "Hearings on the Proposed Transfer of Indian Hospitals and Health Facilities to the Public Health Service," 92, 130-131.

23. *House Report no. 870*, 14. The Committee recommended that the educational responsibilities of the Indian Service be turned over to other agencies serving non-Indians as soon as practicable programs could be worked out. *Congressional Record*, (100), 8959.

24. Oklahoma's delegation included five Democrats (Ed Edmundson, Carl Albert, Tom Steed, John Jarman and Victor Wickersham) and one Republican (Page Belcher). Todd, 7.

25. The Bureau of the Budget requested $125,000 so the Public Health Service could begin the initial steps of transfer before July 1. Letter of Percival F. Brundage, acting Director of the Bureau of the Budget, to the President, March 21, 1955, in "Proposed

Provision-Department of Health, Education and Welfare, Communication for the President of the United States," *Senate Document 16*, 84th Congress, 1st session, March 23, 1955. "Transferring the Maintenance and Operation of Hospitals and Health Services for Indians to the Public Health Service," *House Report no. 2430*, 83rd Congress, 2d session, July 21, 1954. "An Act to transfer the maintenance and operation of hospital and health facilities for Indians to the Public Health Service, and for other purposes," 68 stat 674. *Annual Report of the Secretary of the Interior*, 1955, 231. *Annual Report of the Secretary of Health, Education and Welfare*, 1955, 122.

26. "Labor-Health, Education and Welfare Appropriations for 1959," *Hearings before the Subcommittee of the Committee on Appropriations United States Senate*, 85th Congress, 2d session, April 1, 1958. Shaw argued that more Indians were using the services and that more money was needed to operate the program.

27. *Health Services for American Indians*, 98.

28. Area offices included Portland, Oregon; Aberdeen, South Dakota; Oklahoma City, Oklahoma; Albuquerque, New Mexico; and Phoenix, Arizona. Alaska was setup as an independent area office. Subarea offices were established at Billings, Montana; Bemidji, Minnesota; and Window Rock, Arizona. Both offices operated independently as far as medical and other program supervision was concerned. Area office staff included a medical officer, an assistant medical officer, two graduate nurses, a sanitary engineer, a dental officer, a social worker and several other sundry employees. *Health Services for American Indians*, 98-99.

29. *United States Code of Federal Regulations*, Section 36.12 and Section 36.13, 1956.

30. The Committee's American Indian members included N.B. Johnson, Chief Justice of the Oklahoma Supreme Court; Anna Wauneka, Chair of the Navajo Nation's health committee; and Frank Ducheneaux, Chairman of the Cheyenne River Sioux. Non-Indian members included Robert Atwood (Alaska); Dr. Robert Neff Barr (Minnesota); Former director of the Indian Medical Service, Dr. Fred Foard (North Carolina); Dr. Alexander H. Leighton (New York); Dr. James Perkins (New York); and Dr. Raymond F. Peterson (Montana). "Indian Health Advisory Committee," *Journal of the American Medical Association* (161:6), June 9, 1956, 547. Assistant Indian Commissioner William Zimmerman, Jr., argued if the Public Health Service continued to hold the view that health services were "an act of grace" it was "headed for trouble." William Zimmerman, Jr., "The Role of the Bureau of Indian Affairs," *The Annals of the American Academy of Political and Social Sciences*, May 1957, 37-38.

31. *House Report no. 228*, 84th Congress, 1st session, 12-13. *Health Services for American Indians*, vii.

32. *Health Services for American Indians*, 1. Parron, III-1.

33. *Health Services for American Indians*, 1.

34. *Health Services for American Indians*, 175. "Interior Department Appropriation Bill for 1950," *Hearings before the Subcommittee of the Committee on Appropriations House of Representatives*, 81st Congress, 1st session, part 1, January 26, 1949, 633.

35. *Health Services for American Indians*, 21. Bertram S. Krauss, *Indian Health in Arizona: A Study of Health Conditions among Central and Southern Arizona Tribes* (Tucson: Bureau of Ethnic Research, University of Arizona, 1954), 24.

36. *Health Services for American Indians*, 175. A number of Congressmen inquired of Shaw whether the time could be shortened if Congress appropriated larger amounts of money. Shaw replied it was possible but not probable. "Department of Labor and Health, Education and Welfare Appropriations, 1958," *Hearings before the Subcommittee of the Committee on Appropriations House of Representatives* 85th Congress, 1st session, February 18, 1957, 675-688.

37. *Health Services for American Indians*, 3.

38. Metcalf introduced S. 2021 and Anderson introduced HR 2380. "Constructing Indian Hospitals," *House Report no. 574*, 85th Congress, 1st session, June 17, 1957, 2. "Construction of Indian Hospitals," *Hearings before the Committee on Interstate and Foreign Commerce House of Representatives on HR 204 and HR 2380*, 85th Congress, 1st session, April 9, 1957. Congress built several joint hospitals prior to this. For example, it enacted emergency legislation to construct a joint use hospital in Bernalillo County, New Mexico, as authorized by the act of October 31, 1949 (63 stat. 1049). "Indian Hospitalization Payments to Bernalillo County, New Mexico," *House Report no. 1052*, 85th Congress, 1st session, August 13, 1957. "Indian Hospitalization Payments to Bernalillo County, New Mexico," *Senate Report no. 992*, 85th Congress, 1st session, August 17, 1957. "Authorizing Funds Available for Construction of Indian Health Facilities to be used to Assist in the Construction of Community Hospitals which will Service Indians and Non-Indians," *Senate Report no. 769*, 85th Congress, 1st session, July 30, 1957, 6.

39. Foard energetically supported the act. "Construction of Indian Hospitals," 11-14. G.D. Carlyle Thompson, Executive Officer and Secretary of the Montana State Board of Health and the Chairman of the Indian Health Council of the Association of State and Territorial Health Officers, and Robert Barr, Executive Officer and Secretary of the Minnesota State Board of Health and a member of the Surgeon General's advisory committee on Indian Health, urged Congress to enact the bill. "An Act to authorize funds available for construction of Indian health facilities to be used to assist in the construction of community hospitals which will serve Indians and non-Indians," 71 stat 370. James R. Shaw, "Historical Development of Indian Health Services," unpublished history of the Indian Health Services, University of Arizona, October 18, 1982.

40. Alan Sorkin, *American Indians and Federal Aid* (Brookings Institute, 1971), 61-62. Twelve Indian hospitals were constructed prior to 1925 and only eleven were accredited. "Authorizing Funds Available for Construction of Indian Health Facilities to be Used to Assist in the Construction of Community Hospitals which will Serve Indians and Non-Indians," 3. "Washington News: Grants for Indian and Non-Indian Hospitals" *Journal of the American Medical Association* (163:16), April 20, 1957, 25.

41. *Plan for Medical Facilities Needed for Indian Health Services* (Washington, DC: Public Health Service, Division of Indian Health, 1958), 19.

42. *Senate Report no. 769*, 2. M.B. Folsom to Lister Hill, Chairman of the Senate Committee on Labor and Public Welfare, "Indian Health Facilities-Funds," *United States Code and Administrative News*, vol. II (Washington, DC: GPO, 1957), 1548. The proportionate sharing of overhead construction and basic operating and equipment costs (i.e.: x-ray facilities, operating rooms, heating facilities, etc.) tended to reduce the per-bed construction costs for both Indian and non-Indian communities involved. By enabling the

Division of Indian Health to participate in joint health ventures, additional health facilities and hospitals were established in or near small Indian and non-Indian communities, both of which were unable to support a facility individually. Folsom correctly viewed the law as an "alternative for carrying out the Public Health Service's responsibility for the conservation of Indian health."

43. *Plan for Medical Facilities Needed for Indian Health Services*, 6-7. "Declaring the Sense of Congress on the Closing of Indian Hospitals," 86th Congress, 2d session, January 19, 1960, 1-2. If the Public Health Service sought to close a hospital, ninety days notice had to be given and no facility was to be closed if it created a shortage of facilities or intensified the shortage in any given area.

44. The Navajo service unit was listed twice to illustrate the high priority for modernizing existing hospitals (rank #2) and the lower priority for residual needs (rank #28). New Public Health Service facilities were constructed in Shiprock, New Mexico (seventy-five beds); Eagle Butte, South Dakota (thirty beds); Sells, Arizona (fifty beds); Gallup, New Mexico (two hundred beds); Keams Canyon, Arizona (thirty-eight beds); Kotzebue, Alaska (fifty-three beds); and San Carlos, Arizona (thirty-six beds). Remodeled hospitals were in Pine Ridge, South Dakota; Rosebud, South Dakota; Browning, Montana; and Whiteriver, Arizona. New hospitals were planned for Crow Agency, Montana; Point Barrow, Alaska (twelve beds); Fort Yates, North Dakota (twenty-seven beds); Phoenix, Arizona (two hundred beds); and Lawton, Oklahoma (eighty beds). "Review of the Indian Health Program," *Hearing before the Subcommittee on Indian Affairs of the Committee on Interior and Insular Affairs House of Representatives*, 88th Congress, 1st session, May 23, 1963, 53. *Annual Report of the Secretary of Health, Education and Welfare*, 1961, 198.

45. *Celebrating Thirty Years of Progress: The Indian Health Service and the Sanitation Facilities Construction Program* (Washington, DC: Indian Health Service, 1989), 8. By 1957, there were eighty sanitarian aides. Shaw asked for additional funds to expand training because their Indian peers "enthusiastically" accepted the aides. *Department of Labor and Health, Education and Welfare Appropriation for 1958, Hearings before the Subcommittee of the Committee on Appropriations House of Representatives*, 85th Congress, 1st session, February 18, 1957, 669.

46. *Indian Health Highlights*, 12. "Amending the Act of August 5, 1954," *Senate Report no. 1876*, 85th Congress, 2d session, July 22, 1958, 2.

47. "Indian Sanitation Facilities," *Senate Report no. 589*, 86th Congress, 1st session, June 29, 1959, 4.

48. *Sanitation Facilities Construction: Project Administration Management*, Part I (Washington, DC: Indian Health Service, Division of Environmental Health, 1986), 1-3. The Elko project was funded because of complaints about unsanitary conditions around the colony, which bordered "one of Elko's better residential districts." The city of Elko had provided ninety days emergency services (water, sewer and disposal) but complained to federal officials that it was a federal responsibility. "Elko Indian Sanitation Facilities," *Hearing before the Subcommittee on Health and Science of the Committee on Interstate and Foreign Commerce House of Representatives*, 85th Congress, 1st session, April 10, 1957, 2. The project was funded under 71 stat. 353.

49. "Indian Sanitation Facilities," 2. These bills were HR 849, HR 966, HR 1338,

HR 1768, HR 1979, HR 2349, HR 2546 and HR 3188. Arthur Fleming to Oren Harris, Chairman of the Committee on Interstate and Foreign Commerce, "Indian Sanitation Facilities," 4. "Amending the Act of August 5, 1954," *Senate Report no. 244*, 86th Congress, 1st session, May 11, 1959.

50. "An Act to amend the act of August 5, 1954, and for other purposes," 73 stat. 267. Albert H. Stevenson, "Sanitary Facilities Construction Program for Indians and Alaska Natives," *Public Health Reports* (76:4) April 1961, 317-322.

51. Fleming to Harris, "Indian Sanitation Facilities." *Indian Health in Arizona*, 18, 24. In the first three fiscal years subsequent to the enactment of Public Law 121, 168 construction projects were authorized, seventy-two of which were completed.

52. *Indian Health Highlights*, xvi.

53. *Indian Health Highlights*, xi. Arthur Fleming, "Indian Health," *Public Health Reports* (74:6, 1959), placed the tuberculosis rate drop at 40% between 1953 and 1957. The decrease among Alaska Natives was 63%.

54. *Indian Health Highlights*, xvi. "Infant Death rate of American Indians Dropped 30% Since 1954," in *Journal of the American Medical Association* (180:11), March 17, 1962, 44.

55. Maurice Sievers and James Marquis reported that biliary or gallstones occurred more frequently among American Indians than non-Indians due to the Indians' greater propensity for diabetes, obesity and early childbearing. Maurice L. Sievers and James R. Marquis, "The Southwestern American Indian's Burden: Biliary Disease," *Journal of the American Medical Association* (182:5), November 3, 1962, 570-572.

56. The Indian Health Program of the United States Public Health Service (Washington, DC: Division of Indian Health, 1963), 16.

57. Fleming, "Indian Health," 521-522.

CHAPTER EIGHT

"If You Knew the Conditions"

When Omaha physician Susan La Flesche-Picotte penned her 1907 letter to Commissioner of Indian Affairs Francis Leupp, explaining "that if you knew the conditions and circumstances to be remedied you would do all you could to remedy them," she hinted at the challenges facing the Indian Service. "[N]ow is the time," she stated, "that [the Indians] need the most help." The Indian Service—while providing sundry medical services—did not have organized medical services in 1907. Physicians were subject to agency superintendents and rarely were their voices heard at the commissioner's level, unless, as La Flesche-Picotte did, they personally wrote to him.[1]

From its inception, the United States regarded Indian tribes as nations with whom it could treaty. In the course of the next century and a quarter (1778-1911), the United States made nearly 450 treaties and agreements with tribal nations, each of which was presented as "the supreme law of the land." While treaties guaranteed funds for physicians or hospitals, the political nuances of government meant that Congress infrequently appropriated the funds to carry out such treaty provisions. Consequently, Indian tribes—having ceded vast acreages to the United States in exchange for promises of enumerated services and financial commitments for their people—not only grew dependent on the federal government for such services (with state and local governments absolving themselves of any responsibility) but they were also subject to the whims of the legislative process and its inherent social and political ideologies. Politically disenfranchised, American Indians were shut out of the governing process. When funds were provided—for example, those made available by the 1921 Snyder Act—they were often based on the moral principle of charity rather than on any legal obligation. This was troublesome, as moral responsibilities are subjective. Thus, while the United States had both legal and moral responsibilities to insure and improve the health of the American Indians, it did not feel bound to appropriate the funds necessary to do so.

The welfare of the American Indians and, later Alaska Natives, was closely tied to, and dependent on, the response of the Congress. American Indians were "a conspicuous but powerless population" who found themselves subject to federal policies and programs deemed beneficial and/or expedient by Congress. None of the programs or policies was suggested, initiated or advocated by Indians. All were in one manner or another presented as the solution of the age-old "Indian problem" by members of Congress or special interest groups. The Indian voice was largely silent.[2]

The result of such disconcerting policies was preventive health care was never a goal of the Indian medical service. Instead, it remained curative and crisis-oriented. Health care was doled out with little or no thought of planning for the real needs of the Indians. Funding was based not on need, but on political influence. Fundamental health issues were rarely addressed, except in periodic studies that pried a few dollars out the federal treasury for specific maladies. With many Indians and Alaska Natives living day-to-day in abject poverty, and in some cases in physical misery, their focus was on survival, not how to influence the legislative process.

As the La Flesche-Picotte letter indicates, the challenges in Indian Country were great, growing more pronounced as American Indians were sequestered on reservations. During the first half of the twentieth century, the Indian medical service made nominal progress in the campaign against ill health. Smallpox was virtually eliminated, trachoma curtailed and tuberculosis reduced with the introduction of antibiotics and advances in medical care. Life expectancy increased, with heart and liver diseases rising as tangible signs that the Indians and Alaska Natives were living long enough to experience geriatric diseases. Better pre-natal and neo-natal care meant lower infant and childhood mortality rates. But, while it no longer operated under the theory "that the Indians would ultimately all die of epidemic diseases," the Indian medical service was woefully unprepared to provide overall care. Diseases by and large eliminated or controlled among non-Indians continued to surface among American Indians and Alaska Natives. As acute illnesses decreased, chronic challenges (such as diabetes) soared, especially after 1945.[3]

Many people assumed (and continue to believe so today) that American Indians and Alaska Natives received "free" health care and therefore had fewer health problems than the rest of the American population. But this was far from reality. While health services appeared to be free, the availability of quality services, proximity of resources, particular health challenges and the "willingness of the government to provide adequate funds to maintain and improve health care" all influenced "access to timely and appropriate care." In the years prior to the Indian transfer act, meager funding prevented the setting of a "strong, comprehensive federal Indian health care policy" and the development of a consistent preventive health program.[4]

The Indian Service was not solely accountable for the resultant poor Indian health services. While it was legislatively charged with conserving the health of the Indians, Congress was also culpable. Congress historically vacillated over whether the Indian Service was a necessary evil or an inefficient bureaucracy. It wavered between the social and cultural incorporation of American Indians and the abolition of tribal government on the one hand and the recognition of self-government and cultural preservation on the other. While recognizing the political sovereignty of Indian tribes during the treaty-making era, Congress adopted the policy of complete and rapid assimilation of the Indians after the end of treaty-making.

Assimilationist policies continued until the 1920s, when in a complete reversal of policy—and the result of concerted criticisms of the Indian Service and its overall failures by sympathetic humanitarians—Congress advanced the idea of recognizing and perpetuating Indian social and political existence. This reversal was reflected in the passage of the Indian Reorganization Act, which explicitly acknowledged and encouraged tribal self-government. Additional laws encouraged the cultural renewal of tribes by promoting arts and crafts and fostering economic development. But such policies were ephemeral. After 1946, Congress returned to policies of assimilation, not vacillating until the Indian Health Transfer Act was *fait accompli*.

Since the Indian Service enforced the policies of Congress it, too, was indecisive at times as to what should be done with the Indians. Every commissioner of Indian affairs prior to 1933 advanced in one form or another the concept of complete cultural assimilation as the Indians only salvation. Charles Burke (1921-1929) argued there was no need to increase funding since the Indian Service would cease to exist as the Indians were integrated into American life. Cato Sells (1913-1921) pressed for issuing certificates of competency to Indians freeing their land from trust restrictions, since he saw the role of the Indian Service as emancipating Indians from federal supervision—even if it meant they were handicapped in competing with non-Indians. Dillon Myer (1950-1953) actively promoted the withdrawal of federal support in favor of state and local services.

It was in this context Indian Service employees labored. While they recognized the overarching goal of assimilation, they were less certain of the means by which to effect it. And more personally, they were at times uncertain how long they might be employed. Such dubiety resulted in a dearth of quality employees. As a result, the Indian Service functioned with less qualified health professionals, meaning the overall care provided was inferior to that elsewhere in the country. Some physicians joined the Indian Service out of medical school. Others joined after being denied entrance into other government departments. Still others surfaced in Indian Country after professional improprieties drove them out of mainstream institutions. Most entered with preconceived notions and stayed only until other government or private agencies hired them. Even when qualified staff was available, the Indian Service failed to offer competitive salaries. Working in inadequate facilities with few amenities and social advantages, most physicians left after a year or two.

While there were concerned medical personnel that did all they could with the limited resources they had, far too many were less-than-qualified or not fully committed to serving the patients under their charge. Part of this is attributed to the geographic and cultural isolation providers experienced in Indian Country. Most resulted from the organizational structure and mentality of the Indian Service. With annual turnover rates 50% or more, medical professionals were not around long enough to grasp the extent of illness. Consequently, they failed to understand the cultural definitions and protocol of treating illness.

On another front, the Indian Service did not provide any incentives for its employees to expand their expertise and understanding of the health issues facing American Indians. This partially resulted from the frequent transfers of employees between agencies but generally resulted from medical staff being denied access to professional development. The importance of continuing education and sharing common challenges and research findings with colleagues should not be underestimated. Such intellectual exchange was not only important to the success of the program but also to the well-being of the Indians. Not until the 1930s—with its invitation to the scientific community to assist in the campaign against ill health—did the Indian Service modify this position. At the same time, Congress authorized extended professional development for physicians, although it was not until the 1940s that medical literature was made available at the local level for health care providers.

La Flesche-Picotte also alluded to Congressional parsimony in her comments to Leupp. Parsimony hampered the health program by denying the necessary human and technical resources needed in the campaign against ill health. The needs were great but the resources and financial commitments were limited, handicapping the medical service and forcing many tribes to rely on charity. It was all too common for Indian patients to be treated with less than adequate supplies and resources. Even when funding was available, medical staff was subject to the authority of agency superintendents. Being subordinate to laymen who failed to grasp the complexities of Indian health needs was frustrating. Funds intended for medical services could be—and were—spent on pet projects of the superintendents instead. It was not unusual for superintendents to complete death certificates and determine causes of death—often based on hearsay or their best judgment. Fred Foard identified this as a contentious issue in 1948, believing all medical and hospital services should be under the authority of a medical supervisor who grasped the intricacies of medicine. While this slowly changed—and Indian health concerns were more prominently reported in the annual reports of the Indian

Service—the dearth of epidemiological statistical collection and analysis added to the difficulties.[5]

Scant funding had the obvious effect of limiting services, which in turn impacted the overall status of Indian health. The more subtle effects were just as damaging. The physical misery and psychological effects of not being of sufficient value to warrant the human and financial resources to maintain a minimal level of health care were real and can still be found among some American Indians today. Congressional vacillation, an unstable health corps, inadequate salaries, lack of professional development, subordination to laymen and Congressional parsimony all taxed an Indian medical service that struggled to provide quality care.

Compounding the lack of resources was the biological attack unleashed upon American Indians by exotic diseases. The epidemiological exchange decimated tribes, with mortality rates of 90% or more in the initial years of contact. Having no immunity to contagious diseases, such as smallpox, measles, cholera, scarlet fever and others, the Indians were largely defenseless in resisting epidemics. Successive waves severely handicapped the people, leading to the complete destruction of some tribes.

Lack of immunity and the rapidity of change in the latter nineteenth and early twentieth centuries exposed the Indians to great environmental risks. While the United States was metamorphosing into an industrial nation, such changes were driven by prevailing views of progress, which were accepted and embraced by the westward-moving Americans. For American Indians these changes required physical and cultural adaptations and adjustments, to say nothing of geographic displacement. Because of the rapidity of these changes, American Indians experienced greater challenges that, due to social, cultural and economic pressures, resulted in impoverished environmental conditions. These conditions (poverty, social neglect, contaminated water sources, lack of waste disposal, etc.) compounded disease and poor health.

Environmental variables were further impacted by incoherent and asynchronic government policies. Since the Indian Service was concerned with, and responsible for, social and economic matters, education, land and resource development, and law and order, environmental health matters were frequently obscured and of little importance. An example of this low priority is the fact the Indian Service dedicated just 0.7% of its total budget for health supplies between 1920 and 1924. There was no budget at all for dealing with environmental risks. With such diverse responsibilities—and considering its chronic shortcomings—it was perhaps unrealistic to expect the Indian Service to fulfill any of its responsibilities well, although it did succeed in carrying out its land policies. Between 1887 and 1934 it worked to reduce Indian land holdings from 138,000,000 acres to 48,000,000. In the process, valuable resources the Indians might have used to their economic improvement were removed, adding to the environmental and social woes in Indian Country. The Indian Service assumed, as

Lewis Meriam opined in 1928, that land severalty and private ownership with all of its appurtenant rights and responsibilities would in and of themselves integrate the Indians into American life. Land ownership neither ensured assimilation nor guaranteed good health.[6]

The federal government's land, law, education and administrative policies all worked against its health policy. The former were seemingly designed to effect some level of privation, be it economic, political, cultural or social. The loss of land, political disenfranchisement, cultural disorientation and bureaucratic red tape added to the already monumental environmental and social challenges in Indian Country. Since disease strikes hardest among the poorest, least educated and economically depressed people, health care, including environmental health, should have been the primary function of the Indian Service. Having been sequestered on reservations and subjected to all of the incumbent social and economic ills associated with rapid change, most Indians lived in destitute conditions. The government's desire to assimilate them without taking adequate steps to ensure their health and well-being resulted in high rates of poverty and social decay. Dietary changes and malnutrition further hampered matters. The loss of traditional economies was devastating.[7]

With some exceptions during the 1930s and 1940s, the Indian medical service did not concern itself with the cultural compatibility of its services. While it occasionally brought in a medicine man at the dedication of a hospital, no real effort was made to integrate the Indian conception of health care. J. L. Neave, a former agency physician at the Ft. Berthold (North Dakota) Reservation, expressed the views of many physicians. "These medicine men were now supplied with medicine possessing virtues to heal all the ills that flesh is heir to. And it didn't cost them like it does the modern physician, who has to depend on the manufacturing druggist for his supplies. Neither does your Indian medicine man have to label his medicines. It seems entirely immaterial from what pocket he draws his supplies for the treatment of any given case. The effect of one is just as good as another."[8]

The care and services provided by the Indian medical service were straightforward. Physicians believed they had the cures and the Indians needed them. If Indians sought treatment it was on the terms of the providers. Indians could either adapt to Western views and treatment or forgo services. While many Indians accepted such care, most did so with reservations or as a last resort. Many recognized traditional medicine was ineffective in dealing with the deadly infectious and communicable diseases but they expected some semblance of respect and dignity for their cultural convictions. Dr. Charles Eastman, a Santee Sioux physician, expressed such a view in 1919, when he wrote Indian medicine men "never lost sight of the spiritual side of health and disease" as their non-Indian counterparts did.[9]

By superimposing a foreign health care system over Indian Country without considering the deep-rooted cultural views and considerations of American

Indians and Alaska Natives, the Indian Service effectively precluded itself from operating a medical program that was conducive to the needs of its constituents. While cultural considerations were of minimal concern to the Indian Service, they were a significant indicator of health care acceptance. Failure to consider tribal conceptions of health and well-being doomed most efforts to establish community-based health programs. While the roots of modern day community health programs began in the 1930s, the Indian Service was unable to replicate such programs in Indian Country until after 1950.

The inability to understand or consider how the Indians viewed and defined medical care and treatment further taxed the Indian medical service. Lack of understanding, combined with an attitude of the supremacy of Western medicine to the complete exclusion of Indian conceptions of health, manifested itself in a manner that relegated health care to a secondary concern. Popular and frequent Indian Service critic Haven Emerson hinted at the results of such views when he wrote nowhere in America was the gap between medical knowledge and application as great as in Indian Country. "Any pride this country may feel about its steadily improving health records," Emerson concluded, "must be streaked with shame at these dark spots of shockingly high incidence of sickness and death."[10]

While humanitarians saw education as the key to Indian independence and well-being, few saw the importance of health care and fewer still considered health a fundamental need. One progressive reformer who did was Dr. C. A. Harper, Health Officer for the State of Wisconsin. In 1933, Harper argued health care was more basic than even education and industry. "Take as many whites as there are Indians and give them as much sickness as the Indian has been having," Harper opined, "and the whites would soon be poverty stricken, ambitionless, and immoral. The sicker the Indian gets the worse he lives. Health is the basis of all life." Harper clearly recognized cultural conceptions of health formed the basis of its acceptance.[11]

Not surprisingly, many American Indians remained skeptical and suspicious of Western medicine. Some tenaciously held onto traditional ways of healing and treatment, even though such measures had little or no effect on the diseases ravaging Indian Country. But while having limited effects on disease, the manner in which such services were rendered was culturally sensitive and considered the broader context of health. Western medicine frequently failed to recognize these matters. Cultural taboos were commonly violated. Among the Navajo, for instance, speaking with relatives of the deceased within the four-day period of mourning was a frequently violated taboo.[12]

Among those considered traditionalists, resistance to health services was more frequent, no matter how well intentioned or beneficial such efforts may have been. Such was the case among the Hopi during a smallpox epidemic in 1899. Traditionalists refused vaccinations and disregarded orders of quarantine and fumigation, resulting in the spread of the disease throughout the mesa top villages. Before it was arrested, 74% of the traditionalists were dead while just 6% of those who were vaccinated died.[13]

The outbreak of smallpox among the Hopi also exemplified the cultural insensitivities of government agents and physicians. The bodies of those who died were cremated, rather than buried, in violation of Hopi ways. When Indian agent George W. Hayzlett fumigated homes and clothing, the Hopi were subjected to humiliating disinfectants from strangers and forced to live in temporary camps away from their villages. As a final measure of disgrace, Hayzlett called in thirty federal troops to force the measures on Second Mesa. These insensitivities added to the crisis, as many of the people were convinced that all government efforts were intended to destroy their culture.[14]

Such insensitivity points to an on-going challenge of looking beyond simple cures and corrective measures. In order for health care to be meaningful, the health provider must consider what is culturally relevant. What the Indian Service needed was a paradigm shift. Rather than relegate cultural factors to the background, the Indian Service needed to bring them to the fore. A standard clinical model, such as the crisis-oriented, hospital-based physician services of the Indian medical service, may have been simple and easy to use but it could not factor in cultural norms, customs and traditions.

The implementation of a social conservation model was necessary since it takes into account the life circumstances of the local community and the salient features of community norms. These can then be factored into the medical paradigm, giving it a level of cultural inclusion not considered by the Indian Service. By so doing, statistics such as causes of death, which are easily identified but provide little in terms of guiding research in combating problems, can play a more significant role in determining solutions that are culturally based.[15]

The Indian medical service also needed to consider the art of medicine, not just its science. Providers failed to consider the relationship of the patient and his cultural surroundings. This can only be done by understanding the local conception of wellness and illness, respecting that conception, and working within the local support system in the healing process. Failing to do this, a superimposed health care system was viewed as foreign. This may well be the most important lesson to learn in determining why American Indians and Alaska Natives experienced a disproportionate amount of ill health.[16]

While initially unprepared for the biological assault, American Indians were not inherently predisposed to ill health in the latter nineteenth and first half of the twentieth centuries. And while the quality of medical care was clearly inferior, in and of itself quality care would not have prevented ill health. The same can be said of Congressional parsimony. While greater resources would have enabled the campaign against ill health to be more effective, in and of themselves they would not have prevented ill health. A more fundamental consideration might be the failure of Congress and the Indian Service to consider the deep-seated, culture-based conceptions of health care held by American Indians and Alaska Natives.

Failure to recognize the unique cultural norms and values associated with health and well-being limited the effectiveness of the Indian medical service.

Resistance towards such a system of health care was sure to follow. The mediocre job that resulted justified parsimonious appropriations, initiating a cycle of benign neglect. Factor in a long-standing congressional mandate of cultural assimilation and desire to abolish the Indian Service and one begins to see two parallel themes that shed light on the degree and extent of disease in Indian Country. Insufficient funding and a lack of commitment to improving Indian health care (Congress committed additional money in the 1950s only when it served its stated goal of terminating Indian-only services) were compounded by cultural barriers and restrictions. A reverse dialectic undermined both funding and acceptance of services.

Tribes today recognize they can no longer fully rely on the federal government for complete health care, notwithstanding moral and legal obligations. Tribes use other funds, including gaming revenues, to invest in the health and well-being of their people. If a tribe chooses to implement traditional healing practices, it must be free of restrictive federal regulatory control. As tribes and tribal groups come to control the health services of their people, they are in a position to direct policies, procedures and practices that reflect their unique cultural and social realities. The lesson to be learned is that tribes can blend the best of Western medicine (formal Indian Health Service services) with the best of their traditional ways. Only when these dual factors of funding and culture are considered will the discrepancies between Indian and non-Indian health be eliminated.

Notes

1. Handwritten letter from Dr. Susan La Flesche-Picotte to Commissioner of Indian Affairs Francis Leupp.

2. Murray L. Wax, "Educating an Anthro," in Thomas Biolsi and Larry J. Zimmerman, *Indians and Anthropologists: Vine Deloria Jr., and the Critique of Anthropology* (Tucson: University of Arizona Press, 1997), 53.

3. Gregg, 38.

4. Jennie Joe, "The Delivery of Health Care to American Indians: History, Policies and Prospects," in Donald E. Green and Thomas V. Tonnesen, *American Indians: Social Justice and Public Policy* (Milwaukee, Wisconsin: University of Wisconsin System, Institute on Race and Ethnicity, 1991), 150.

5. Some physicians in Alaska arrived at isolated medical facilities only to find obsolete, rusty medical equipment. Personal interview with Dr. Stanley Stitt, retired Public Health Service physician, Tucson, Arizona, February 14, 1990. Braasch, 221. Board of Indian Commissioners, *Annual Report*, 1932, 29

6. Gessner, 237. Meriam, 7.

7. David H. DeJong, "See the New Country: The Removal Controversy and Pima-Maricopa Water Rights, 1869-1879," *The Journal of Arizona History* (33:4, Winter 1992),

367-396. David H. DeJong, "A Scheme to Rob Them of Their Land? Water, Allotment and the Economic Integration of the Pima Reservation, 1902-1921," *The Journal of Arizona History*, (44:2 Summer 2003), 99-132.

8. J.L. Neave, "An Agency Doctor's Experience among Frontier Indians," *Cincinnati Medical Journal*, vol. 9, 1894, 875-876.

9. Charles Eastman, "The Medicine Man's Practice," *Pharmaceutical Era*, vol. 52, 1919, 281.

10. The Indian Service blamed Congressional parsimony for the lack of clerical workers to assist in maintaining even rudimentary records. "Indian Hospitals Rank among Nation's Best," 13-14. Emerson, 219.

11. Quoted in Gessner, 198.

12. "Navajos curtail health studies," *The Arizona Republic* (106:172, November 6, 1995), A-1.

13. Trennert, "White Man's Medicine vs. Hopi Tradition: The Smallpox Epidemic of 1899," 359.

14. Trennert, 360-364.

15. John Red Horse, Troy Johnson and Diane Weiner, "Commentary: Cultural Perspectives on Research among American Indians," *American Indian Culture and Research Journal* (13:3-4, 1989). It would also be meaningful to more closely examine the relationship between quality of care, health promotion and disease prevention. Current research supports the distribution of resources to support secondary and tertiary care rather than the primary cause of ill health. The result is the core problem is never fully addressed.

16. "Tribes urge Western doctors to be more open to 'old ways'," *The Arizona Republic* (104:84, August 9, 1993), A-1.

Bibliography

THE NATIONAL ARCHIVES OF THE UNITED STATES:

Ratified Treaties 1854-1855. National Archives, Record Group 75, Indian Records Office.

Ratified Treaties 1856-1863. National Archives, Record Group 75, Indian Records Office.

Official Letters of W. J. McConnell. National Archives, Record Group 48, Secretary of the Interior Records Office.

Indian Inspection Reports. National Archives, Record Group 48, Office of the Secretary of the Interior, Indian Division.

Office of Indian Affairs, Circulars. National Archives, Record Group 75, Educational Circulars.

GOVERNMENT DOCUMENTS:

American Indian and Alaska Native Population: 2000, United States Department of Commerce, Census Bureau, February 2002.

American Red Cross. "A Study of the Need for Public Health Nursing on Indian Reservations." *Survey of Conditions of the Indians in the United States: Hearings Before a Subcommittee of the Committee on Indian Affairs,* Part 3, 1929.

Board of Indian Commissioners, *Annual Report,* Washington, DC: GPO.

Bureau of Indian Affairs, Branch of Health. *Indian Health: A Problem and a*

Challenge, Washington, DC: GPO, 1955.

Commission on the Organization of the Executive Branch of Government: Functions and Activities of the National Government in the Field of Welfare, Washington, DC: GPO, 1949.

Declaring the Sense of Congress on the Closing of Indian Hospitals, 86th Congress, 2nd session, Public Health Service, Division of Indian Health, 1960.

Federal Register, volume 1, 1936.

Final Report to the American Indian Policy Review Commission, Task Force Six: Report on Indian Health, Washington, DC: GPO, 1976.

Mountin, Joseph W., and James G. Townsend. *Observations on Indian Health Problems and Facilities*, United States Treasury Department, Public Health Service, Public Health Bulletin no. 223, Washington, DC: GPO, 1936.

Murphy, Joseph F. *Manual on Tuberculosis: Its Causes, Prevention and Treatment*, Washington, DC: GPO, 1910.

Newberne, Robert E.L., "A Review of Miss Patterson's Report Entitled 'A Study of the Need for Public Health Nursing on Indian Reservations'," in *A Survey of Conditions of the Indians in the United States: Hearings Before a Subcommittee of the Committee on Indian Affairs*, Part 3, 1929.

Office of Indian Affairs, *Regulations for the Indian Department*. Washington, DC: GPO, 1884.

Office of Indian Affairs. *The Indian Service Health Activities*, Bulletin 11, Washington, DC: GPO, 1922.

Regional Differences in Indian Health, 1998-1999, Washington, DC: Public Health Service, Indian Health Service, 2000.

Sanitation Facilities Construction: Project Administration and Management, Part 1. Washington, DC: Indian Health Service, Division of Environmental Health, 1986.

Secretary of Health, Education and Welfare. *Annual Report*, Washington, DC: GPO.

Secretary of the Interior. *Annual Report*, Washington, DC: GPO.

Statutes at Large of the United States of America, 1789-1873, 17 volumes. Washington, DC: GPO.

Bibliography

167

United States Bureau of Indian Affairs. *Annual Report of the Commissioner of Indian Affairs*, Washington, DC: GPO.

United States Code and Administrative News, 83rd Congress, 1st session, Washington, DC: GPO, 1954.

United States Code of Federal Regulations, Washington, DC: GPO, 1956.

United States Congressional Record, Washington, DC: GPO.

United States Congress. House. *Smallpox among the Indians, Letter from the Secretary of War upon the Subject of the Small Pox among the Indian tribes.* 22nd Congress, 1st session, 1832. H. Doc. 190.

United States Congress. House. *Letter From the Secretary of War, Transmitting a Report of the Commissioner of Indian Affairs in relation to the execution of the act extending the benefit of Vaccination to the Indian Tribes, &c.* 22nd Congress, 2nd session, 1833. H. Doc. 82.

United States Congress. House. *Smallpox among the Indians, Letter from the Secretary of War upon the Subject of the Small Pox among the Indian tribes.* 25th Congress, 3rd session, 1838. H. Doc. 51.

United States Congress. House. *Conditions of Reservation Indians, Letter from the Secretary of the Interior*, 57th Congress, 1st session, 1901. H. Doc. 406.

United States Congress. House. *To Provide for Compulsory Education of Native Children of Alaska, and for the Enforcement of Sanitary Regulations among the Natives of Alaska.* 60th Congress, 1st session, 1908. H. Rep. 1372.

United States Congress. House. *Report on the Matter of the Investigation of the Indian Bureau with Transcripts of Testimony Taken and Exhibits offered from April 9, 1912 to August 17, 1912*, 62nd Congress, 3rd session, 1913. H. Rep. 1279.

United States Congress. House. *Report of the Joint Commission on Indian Tuberculosis Sanitarium and Yakima Indian Reservation Project.* 63rd Congress, 2nd session, 1915. H. Doc. 505.

United States Congress. House. Committee on Indian Affairs. *Letter from Secretary of the Interior to the House Committee on Indian Affairs.* 63rd Congress, 2nd session, 1915. H. Doc. 1254.

United States Congress. House. Committee on Indian Affairs. *Indians of the United States: Hearings Before the Committee on Indian Affairs on the Condition of Various Tribes of Indians.* 66th Congress, 1st session, 1919.

United States Congress. House. *Reorganizing the Indian Service.* 66th Congress,

3rd session, 1919. H. Rep. 1189.

United States Congress. House. *Reorganizing the Indian Service: Report of the Committee of Indian Affairs.* 67th Congress, 1st session, 1921. H. Rep. 1278.

United States Congress. House. *Reorganizing the Indian Service: Report of the Committee of Indian Affairs.* 67th Congress, 1st session, 1921. H. Rep. 1228.

United States Congress. House. *The Indian Problem: Resolution of the Committee of One Hundred appointed by the Secretary of the Interior and a Review of the Indian Problem.* 68th Congress, 1st session, 1924. H. Doc. 149.

United States Congress. House. *Hearings on H.R. 8821.* 69th Congress, 1st session, 1926.

United States Congress. House. *Subcommittee of the Committee on Indian Affairs, Hearings before the Subcommittee on General Bills of the Committee on Indian Affairs.* 74th Congress, 1st session, 1935. House Bill 7781.

United States Congress. House. Committee on Appropriations. *Hearings on the Indian Appropriation Act of 1939,* Washington, DC: GPO, 1939.

United States Congress. House. *Interior Department Appropriation Bill for 1950: Hearings before the Subcommittee of the Committee on Appropriations.* 81st Congress, 1st session, 1949.

United States Congress. House. *Transfer the Maintenance and Operation of Hospitals and Health Facilities for Indians to the Public Health Service.* 83rd Congress, 1st session, 1953. H. Rep. 870.

United States Congress. House. *Transferring the Maintenance and Operation of Hospitals and Health Services for Indians to the Public Health Service.* 83rd Congress, 2nd session. H. Rep. 2430.

United States Congress. House. 84th Congress, 1st session, 1954. H. Rep. 228.

United States Congress. House. *Elko Indian Sanitation Facilities, Hearings before the Subcommittee on Health and Science of the Committee on Interstate and Foreign Commerce.* 85th Congress, 1st session, 1957.

United States Congress. House. *Department of Labor and Health, Education and Welfare Appropriations, 1958: Hearings before the Subcommittee of the Committee on Appropriations, House of Representatives.* 85th Congress, 1st session, 1957.

United States Congress. House. *Constructing Indian Hospitals.* 85th Congress, 1st session, 1957. H. Rep. 574.

United States Congress. House. *Constructing Indian Hospitals, Hearings before the Committee on Interstate and Foreign Commerce, House of Representatives on HR 204 and HR 2380.* 85th Congress, 1st session, 1957.

United States Congress. House. *Indian Hospitalization Payments to Bernalillo County, New Mexico.* 85th Congress, 1st session, 1957. H. Rep. 1052.

United States Congress. House. *Review of Indian Health Program, Hearings before the Subcommittee on Indian Affairs of the Committee on Interior and Insular Affairs.* 88th Congress, 1st session, 1963.

United States Congress. Senate. *Memorial of Sylvanus Fansher praying for the Establishment of a permanent vaccine institute for the benefit of the army, navy and Indian Department.* 25th Congress, 3rd session, 1838. S. Doc. 385.

United States Congress. Senate. *Condition of the Indian Tribes: Report of the Joint Special Committee appointed under Joint Resolution of March 3, 1865.* 39th Congress, 2nd session, 1867. S. Rep. 156.

United States Congress. Senate. *Trachoma in Certain Indian Schools.* 60th Congress, 2nd session, 1909. S. Rep. 1025.

United States Congress. Senate. *For Relief of Certain Indians: Letter from the Secretary of the Treasury.* 61st Congress, 1st session, 1909. S. Doc. 148.

United States Congress. Senate. *Trachoma in Certain Indian Schools.* 62nd Congress, 2nd session, 1911. S. Rep. 1025.

United States Congress. Senate. *Diseases among the Indians: Message from the President of the United States in Relation to the present Conditions of Health on Indian Reservations and in Indian Schools.* 62nd Congress, 2nd session, 1912. S. Doc. 907.

United States Congress. Senate. *Memorial of the Brotherhood of North American Indians.* 62nd Congress, 2nd session, 1912. S. Doc. 489.

United States Congress. Senate. *Diseases among the Indians: A Letter from the Acting Secretary of the Treasury transmitting a copy of a letter from the Secretary of the Interior, August 14, 1912.* 62nd Congress, 2nd session, 1912. S. Doc. 920.

United States Congress. Senate. *Contagious and Infectious Diseases among the Indians.* 62nd Congress, 3rd session, 1913. S. Doc. 1038.

United States Congress. Senate. *Committee on Indian Affairs, Tuberculosis among the North American Indians: Report of a Committee of the National Tuberculosis Association.* 67th Congress, 4th Session, 1923.

United States Congress. Senate. *Hearings on S 3020.* 69th Congress, 1st session, 1926.

United States Congress. Senate. Subcommittee of the Committee on Indian Affairs, *Survey of Conditions of the Indians in the United States: Hearings Before a Subcommittee of the Committee on Indian Affairs.* 1929-1942.

United States Congress, Senate. S. Rep. 511, 73rd Congress, 2nd session, 1934.

United States Congress. Senate. *Survey of Conditions among the Indians.* 78th Congress, 2nd session, 1945. S. Rep. 310.

United States Congress. Senate. *Aspects of Indian Policy.* 79th Congress, 1st session, 1945.

United States Congress, Senate. *Rehabilitation of the Navajo and Hopi Indians: Hearings Before a Subcommittee on Interior and Insular Affairs in the United States Senate.* 80th Congress. 2nd session, 1948.

United States Congress. Senate. *Providing for Medical Services for Non-Indians in Indian Hospitals.* 81st Congress, 1st session, 1949. S. Rep. 1095.

United States Congress. Senate. *Transfer of Indian Hospitals and Health Facilities to Public Health Service: Hearings Before a Subcommittee of the Committee on Interior and Insular Affairs on H.R. 303.* 83rd Congress, 2nd session, 1954.

United States Congress. Senate. *Hearings on the Proposed transfer of Indian Hospitals and Health Facilities to the Public Health Service, Hearings before the Committee on Interior and Insular Affairs, US Senate.* 83rd Congress, 2nd session, 1954.

United States Congress. Senate. *Proposed Provision—Department of Health, Education and Welfare, Communication for the President of the United States.* 84th Congress, 1st session. 1955. S. Doc. 16.

United States Congress. Senate. *Urgent Deficiencies Appropriation Bill 1956: Hearings before the Committee on Appropriations, US Senate on H.R. 9063.* 84th Congress, 2nd session, 1956.

United States Congress. Senate. *Indian Hospitalization Payments to Bernalillo County, New Mexico.* 85th Congress, 1st session, 1957.

United States Congress. Senate. *Authorizing Funds Available for Construction of Indian Health Facilities to be used to Assist in the Construction of Community Hospitals which will Service Indians and Non-Indians.* 85th Session, 1st session, 1957. S. Rep. 769.

United States Congress. Senate. *Amending the Act of August 5, 1954.* 85th

Congress, 2nd session, 1958. S. Rep. 1876.

United States Congress. Senate. *Labor-Health, Education and Welfare Appropriation for 1959, Hearings before the Subcommittee of the Committee on Appropriations.* 85th Congress, 2nd session, 1958.

United States Congress. Senate. *Indian Sanitation Facilities.* 86th Congress, 1st session, 1959. S. Rep. 589.

United States Congress. Senate. *Amending the Act of August 5, 1954.* 86th Congress, 1st session, 1959. S. Rep. 244.

United States Department of Health, Education and Welfare. *A Study of the Indian Health Service and Tribal Involvement in Health.* Prepared by Urban Associates, Washington, DC: GPO, 1974.

United States Department of Health, Education and Welfare. *Indian Health Highlights.* Washington, DC: GPO, 1964.

United States Department of Health, Education and Welfare, Public Health Service. *Health Services for American Indians.* Washington, DC: GPO, 1957.

United States Department of Health, Education and Welfare, Public Health Service, Division of Indian Health. *Plan for Medical Facilities Needed for Indian Health Services.* Washington, DC: GPO, 1958.

United States Department of Health and Human Services, Public Health Service, Indian Health Service. *Celebrating Thirty Years of Progress: The Indian Health Service and the Indian Sanitation Facilities Construction Program.* Washington, DC: GPO, 1989.

United States Statutes at Large, 1874-1959. Washington, DC: GPO.

COURT DECISIONS:

A Matter of Heff, 197 U.S. Reports 488, (1905).

Harrison v. Laveen, 196 Pacific Reporter 456 (1948).

Status of Alaskan Natives, 52 Decisions of the Department of the Interior 597 (1929).

Status of Alaskan Natives, 53 Decisions of the Department of the Interior 593 (1932).

United States v. Lynch, 7 Alaska Reports 568 (1927).

United States v. Nice, 241 United States Reports 591 (1916).

BOOKS:

Boyd, Robert. *The Coming of the Spirit of Pestilence.* Vancouver: University of British Columbia Press, 1999.

Collier, John. *From Every Zenith.* Denver, Colorado: Swallow Publishing, 1963.

Crosby, Alfred W. *The Columbian Exchange.* Westport, CT: Greenwood Publishing Company, 1972.

DeJong, David H. *Promises of the Past: A History of Indian Education.* Golden, Colorado: North American Press, 1993.

Dobyns, Henry F., and William R. Swagerty. *Their Number Became Thinned.* Knoxville: University of Tennessee Press, 1983.

Fixico, Donald L. *Termination and Relocation: Federal Indian Policy 1945-1960.* Albuquerque: University of New Mexico Press, 1986.

Foreman, Grant. *Indian Removal.* Norman: University of Oklahoma Press, 1932.

Gessner, Robert. *Massacre: A Survey of Today's American Indians.* New York: Jonathan Cape and Harrison Smith, 1931.

Gregg, Elinor D. *The Indian and the Nurse.* Norman: University of Oklahoma Press, 1965.

Iverson, Peter. *Carlos Montezuma and the Changing World of American Indians.* Albuquerque: University of New Mexico Press, 1982.

Kelly, Lawrence C. *The Navaho Indians and Federal Indian Policy.* Tucson: University of Arizona Press, 1968.

Krauss, Bertram S. *Indian Health in Arizona: A Study of Health Conditions among Central and Southern Arizona Tribes.* Tucson: University of Arizona, Bureau of Ethnic Research, 1954.

LaFarge, Oliver. *The Changing Indian.* Norman: University of Oklahoma Press, 1942.

Meriam, Lewis. *The Problem of Indian Administration.* Baltimore: John Hopkins Press, 1928.

Moorhead, Warren K. *The American Indians in the United States: 1850-1914*. Freeport, New York: Books for Liberty Press, 1969 reprint.

Parron, Thomas. *Alaska's Health: A Survey*. The Graduate School of Public Health, University of Pittsburgh, 1954.

Philp, Kenneth R. *John Collier's Crusade for Indian Reform: 1920-1954*. Tucson: University of Arizona Press, 1977.

Prucha, Francis Paul. *The Great Father: The United States Government and the American Indians*, volume 2. Lincoln: University of Nebraska Press, 1986.

—— *American Indian Policy in the Formative Years: The Indian Trade and Intercourse Acts, 1790-1834*. Lincoln: University of Nebraska Press, 1962.

Raup, Ruth. *The Indian Health Program 1800-1955*. Washington, DC: GPO, 1959.

Schmeckebier, Laurence F. *The Office of Indian Affairs: Its History, Activities and Organization*. Baltimore: John Hopkins Press, 1927.

Sorkin, Alan. *American Indians and Federal Aid*. Brookings Institute, 1971.

Schoolcraft, Henry Rowe. *Information Respecting the History, Conditions and Prospects of the Indian Tribes of the United States*, volume 1. Philadelphia, 1853.

Thornton, Russell. *American Indian Holocaust and Survival: A Population Study Since 1492*. Norman: University of Oklahoma Press, 1987.

Townsend, James G. "Indian Health-Past, Present and Future," in Oliver LaFarge, ed. *The Changing Indian*. Norman: University of Oklahoma Press, 1942.

Transactions of the Sixth International Congress on Tuberculosis. Philadelphia: William F. Fall, 1908.

Trennert, Robert. *The Phoenix Indian School: Forced Assimilation in the Desert, 1891-1935*. Norman: University of Oklahoma Press, 1988.

Vogel, Virgil J. *American Indian Medicine*. Norman: University of Oklahoma Press, 1970.

Washburn, Wilcomb E. *The Indian in America*. New York: Harper and Row, 1975.

ARTICLES:

—— *Indian Truth* 8 (1931).

—— *Indians at Work* 8:5 (1941)

Adair, John, Kurt Deuschle and Walsh McDermott. "Patterns of Health and Disease among the Navahoes." *The Annals of the American Academy of Political and Social Science* 311 (1957).

Adair, John and Kurt Deuschle. "Some Problems of the Physicians on the Navajo Reservation." *Human Organization* 16:4 (1958).

"Aleut Hospital at Unalaska destroyed by Japanese Bombs." *Indians at Work* 10:1 (1942).

Allen, A. R. "Hospital Management and the Training of Indian Girls as Nurses." *The Red Man* 4:2 (1911).

"A.M.A. Leaders and Secretary Krug Plan New Medical Missions." *Journal of the American Medical Association* 139:14 (1949).

Aronson, Joseph D. "Appraisal of Protective Value of BCG Vaccine." *Journal of the American Medical Association* 149:4 (1952).

Aronson, Joseph D., and Helen C. Taylor. "The Trend of Tuberculous Infections among some Indian Tribes and the Effectiveness of BCG Vaccination on Tuberculin Testing." *The American Review of Tuberculosis and Pulmonary Disease* 72 (1955).

Beatty, Willard. "Uncle Sam Develops a New Kind of Rural School." *Elementary School Journal* 41 (1940).

Benson, Otis O. "Conditions in the Indian Medical Service." *Journal of the American Medical Association* 81:16 (1923).

Braasch, W.F., B.J. Branton and A.J. Chesley. "Survey of Medical Care among the Upper Midwest Indians." *Journal of the American Medical Association* 139:4 (1949).

Breid, Jacob. "East Farm Sanatorium School." *The Red Man* 6:9 (1914).

Collier, John. *American Indian Life* April, 1934.

—— "The Red Atlantis." *Survey* 49:10 (1922).

—— "Health Program of the Indian Service." *Indians at Work* 9:6 (March-April, 1944).

"Committee on Legislation." *Journal of the American Medical Association* 149:3

(1952).

"Committee on Legislation." *Journal of the American Medical Association* 151:9 (1953).

"Committee on Legislation." *Journal of the American Medical Association* 152:2 (1953).

"Committee on Legislation." *Journal of the American Medical Association* 155:8 (1954).

"Community Meeting on Health Problems at the New Salt River Day School, Arizona." *Indians at Work* 3:24 (1936).

Cook, Sherburne F. "Disease and Extinction of New England Indians." *Human Biology* 45:3 (1973).

—— "The Epidemic of 1830-1833 in California and Oregon." *University of California Publications in American Archaeology and Ethnology* (1950).

Crosby, Alfred W. "Virgin Soil Epidemics as a Factor in the Aboriginal Depopulation in America." *William and Mary Quarterly* 3:33 (1976).

Davis, Burnet M. "The Health Program of the Bureau of Indian Affairs." *The Military Surgeon* 112:3 (March 1953).

DeJong, David H. "See The New Country: The Removal Controversy and Pima-Maricopa Water Rights, 1869-1879." *The Journal of Arizona History* 33:4 (1992).

—— "A Scheme to Rob them of their Land? Water, Allotment and the Economic Integration of the Pima Reservation, 1902-1921." *The Journal of Arizona History* 44:2 (2003).

DeKruif, Paul. "They Wait for Light." *Country Gentlemen* (1940).

DeLien, H. and J. Nixon Hadley. "How to Recognize an Indian Health Problem." *Human Organization* 11:3 (1952).

Dobyns, Henry F. "Native Historic Epidemiology in the Greater Southwest." *American Anthropologist* 91:1 (1989).

Donehoo, George P. "The White Plague of the Red Man." *The Red Man* 5:1 (1913).

"Dr. Joseph David Aronson appointed Special Expert on Tuberculosis." *Journal of the American Medical Association* 105:14 (1935).

"Drama in the Life of Indian Field Nurses." *Indians at Work* 2:22 (1935).

Endersbee, William. "Soil Conservation on Indian Lands." *Indians at Work* (1945).

Emerson, Haven. "Morbidity of the American Indians." *Science* 68:1626 (1926).

—— "Health of American Indians." *Journal of the American Medical Association* 88:13 (1927).

—— "Indian Health-Victim of Neglect." *The Survey* 87:5 (1951).

Fleming, Arthur. "Indian Health." *Public Health Reports* 74:6 (1959).

Foard, Fred. "The Health of the American Indians." *American Journal of Public Health* 39:11 (1949).

—— "The Federal Government and the American Indian's Health." *Journal of the American Medical Association* 142:5 (1950).

Forster, Wesley G. "Trachoma." *American Journal of Ophthalmology* 27:10 (1944).

—— "Treatment of Trachoma with Sulfanilamide." *American Journal of Ophthalmology* 23:5 (1940).

Fox, Webster L. "Conditions in the Indian Medical Service." *Journal of the American Medical Association* 81:18 (1923).

"George Frazier Wins Achievement Medal." *Indians at Work* 8:4 (1939).

"Government Services." *Journal of the American Medical Association* 152:14 (1953).

"Government Services: Public Health Service." *Journal of the American Medical Association* 160:7 (1956).

Gradle, Harry S. "Abstract of Discussion." *Journal of the American Medical Association* 111:15 (1938).

Gregg, Elinor D. "Indian Nurses Receive Training in Rural Health Work in Frontier Nursing Service." *Indians at Work* 2:15 (1935).

—— "Nursing Care for Indians-Yesterday and Today." *Indians at Work* 4:4 (1936).

Guthrie, Marshall C. "Health of American Indians." *Journal of the American Medical Association* 88:15 (1927).

Hadley, J. Nixon. "Health Conditions among Navaho Indians." *Public Health Reports* 70:9 (1955).

"Health Program of the Indian Service." *Indians at Work* 9:6 (1944).

Hoffman, Fredrick L. "Conditions in the Indian Medical Service." *Journal of the American Medical Association* 75:7 (1920).

—— "Conditions in the Indian Medical Service." *Journal of the American Medical Association* 81:10 (1923).

Hrdlicka, Ales. "Disease, Medicine, and Surgery among the American Aborigines." *Journal of the American Medical Association* 99:20 (1932).

—— "Tuberculosis among Certain Indian Tribes of the United States." *Bureau of American Ethnology* Bulletin 42, Washington, DC: GPO, (1909).

—— "The Vanishing Indian." *Science* 46:1185 (1917).

"Indian Health Advisory Committee." *Journal of the American Medical Association* 161:6 (1956).

"Indian Hospitals Rank among Nation's Best." *Indians at Work* 9:6 (1942).

"Indian Service Hospitals Gradually Meeting Standards for Acceptance by the American College of Surgeons." *Indians at Work* 5:2 (1937).

"Infant Death Rate of American Indians Dropped 30% Since 1954." *Journal of the American Medical Association* 180:11 (1962).

"Influenza Among American Indians." *Public Health Reports* 34 (1919).

Jean, Sally Lucas, "Health Institute." *Indians at Work* 3:4 (1935).

Joe, Jennie, "The Delivery of Health Care to American Indians: History, Policies and Prospects." in Donald E. Green and Thomas V. Tonnesen, eds. *American Indians: Social Justice and Public Policy*. Milwaukee: University of Wisconsin System, Institute on Race and Ethnicity, 1991.

Julianelle, L.A, M.C. Morris and R.W. Harrison, "Studies on the infectivity of trachoma: Further observations on the filterability of the infectious agent." *American Journal of Ophthalmology* 20 (1937).

Leupp, Francis. "Outlines of an Indian Policy." *Outlook* 79 (1905).

"Lifting the Shadows." *Indians at Work* 8:9 (1941).

Loe, Fred. "Sulfanilamide Treatment of Trachoma." *Journal of the American Medical Association* 111:15 (1938).

Marcus, Fanny T. "Public Health Nursing." *Indians at Work* 2:16 (1935).

Matthews, Washington. "Consumption among the Indians." *Transactions of the American Climatological Association.* (1886).

—— "Further Contribution to the Study of Consumption among the Indians." *Transactions of the American Climatological Association.* (1886).

"McGibony Named Director of Health of Indian Service." *Journal of the American Medical Association* 117:2 (1941).

McKay, Mary. "The Rosebud Sioux organize for Health." *Indians at Work* 4:8 (1944).

"Medical News." *Journal of the American Medical Association* 104:8 (1935).

"Medical News." *Journal of the American Medical Association* 106:2 (1936).

"Medical News." *Journal of the American Medical Association* 107:18 (1936).

"Medical News." *Journal of the American Medical Association* 109:13 (1937).

"Medical News." *Journal of the American Medical Association* 113:13 (1939).

"Medical News." *Journal of the American Medical Association* 115:11 (1940).

"Medical News." *Journal of the American Medical Association* 150:16 (1952).

Meritt, Edgar, "Sanitary Homes for Indians." *The Red Man* 4:10 (1912).

—— "Health Conditions among the Indians." *The Red Man* 6:9 (1914).

Moorman, Lewis. "Health of the Navajo-Hopi Indians." *Journal of the American Medical Association* 139:6 (1949).

Murphy, Joseph F. "The Prevention of Tuberculosis in the Indian Schools." *Journal of Proceedings and Addresses of the Forty-Seventh Annual Meeting.* Winona, Minnesota: National Education Association (1909).

—— "Health Problems of the Indians." *The Annals of the American Academy of*

Political and Social Science 37:2 (1911).

"Nature of Filterable Agent of Trachoma." *Journal of the American Medical Association* 111:20 (1938).

"New Director Appointed for Indian Medical Service." *Indians at Work* 8:10 (1941).

"New Director of Indian Health." *Journal of the American Medical Association* 138:6 (1948).

Newton, Elsie E. "The Going Home Women." *The Red Man* 6:9 (1914).

Old, H. Norman. "Sanitation Problems of the American Indians." *The American Journal of Public Health* 43 (1953).

"Organizational News." *Journal of the American Medical Association* 149:3 (1952).

Owens, William B., Ralph F. Honess and James R. Simon. "Protozoal Infestations of American Indian Children." *Journal of the American Medical Association* 102:12 (1934).

Red Horse, John, Troy Johnson and Diane Weiner, "Commentary: Cultural Perspective on Research among American Indians." *American Indians Culture and Research Journal* 13:3-4 (1989).

Salo, Wilmar L., Arthur C. Aufderheide, Jane Buikstra, and Todd A. Holcomb. "Identification of Mycobacterium Tuberculosis DNA in a pre-Columbian Peruvian Mummy." *Proceedings of the National Academy of Science* 91:6 (1994).

Sanders, Rosella. "Indian Medical Service Pioneers in Trachoma Treatment." *Indians at Work* 8:4 (1940).

Sievers, Maurice and James Marquis, "The Southwest American Indian Burden: Biliary Disease." *Journal of the American Medical Association* 182:5 (1962).

Snow, Dean R., and William A. Starna. "Sixteenth Century Depopulation: A View From the Mohawk Valley." *American Anthropologist* 91:1 (1989).

Stevenson, Albert, "Sanitation Facilities Construction Program for Indians and Alaska Natives." *Public Health Reports* 76:4 (1961).

"The Indians' Health and Public Health." *American Journal of Public Health* 44 (1954).

"The Institute for Training Navajo Nurses Aides." *Indians at Work* 1:21 (1934).

"The Rosebud Sioux Organize for Health." *Indians at Work* 4:8 (1944).

Thygeson, Phillips, "The Treatment of Trachoma with Sulfanilamide." *American Journal of Ophthalmology* 23:6 (1940).

——, and F.I. Proctor, "Filterability of Trachoma Virus." *Archives of Ophthalmology* 13 (1930).

——, and Polk Richards, "Etiologic Significance of the elementary body in trachoma." *American Journal of Ophthalmology* 18 (1935).

Townsend, James G. "Health Activities in Alaska." *Indians at Work* 4:4 (1936).

—— "Trachoma, Dreaded Eye Disease, Being Conquered." *Indians at Work* 7:4 (1939).

—— "Special Trachoma Advisory Committee holds first Meeting." *Indians at Work* 4:6 (1937).

—— "The Battle against Tuberculosis Goes Forward." *Indians at Work* 6:8 (1934).

"Trachoma Eradication." *Science* 90:2341, Supplement 10 (1939).

Trennert, Robert A. "White Man's Medicine vs. Hopi Tradition: The Smallpox Epidemic of 1899." *Journal of Arizona History* 33:4, 1992.

"Tuberculosis among the Indians." *Indians at Work* 3:8 (1935).

"Washington News." *Journal of the American Medical Association* 158:11 (1955).

"Washington News: Grants for Indian and Non-Indian Hospitals." *Journal of the American Medical Association* 163:16 (1957).

Work, Hubert. "Letters to the Editor." *Journal of the American Medical Association* 81 (1923).

Wyman, Leland C. and Flora L. Bailey. "Two Examples of Navaho Physiotherapy." *American Anthropologist* 46:3 (1944).

Zimmerman, Charles L., "An Appeal for Prenatal Care." *The Red Man* 9:7 (1917).

Zimmerman, William Jr., "The Role of the Bureau of Indian Affairs," *The Annals of the Academy of Political and Social Science* (1957).

MISCELLANEOUS:

 Stitt, Stanley (Retired Public Health Service Physician) personal interview, with author, February 14, 1990, Tucson, Arizona.

NEWSPAPERS:

 Arizona Republic, August 9, 1993.

 Arizona Republic, November 6, 1995.

 New York Times, October 17, 1933.

UNPUBLISHED WORKS:

 Sense, Richard. "The Transformation of Chippewa Life on the Red Lake Reservation, Minnesota: 1865-1921." Unpublished research paper, American Indian Studies Department, University of Arizona, 1989.

 Shaw, James R. "Indian Health in Historical Perspective." Unpublished paper courtesy of the author, dated October 18, 1982, Tucson, Arizona.

 ―― "Historical Development of Indian Health Services." Unpublished paper courtesy of the author, dated October 18, 1982, Tucson, Arizona.

 Todd, John. *Interview with Dr. James R. Shaw.* Unpublished Document in the Commissioned Corps Centennial Archives, History of Medicine Division, Library of Medicine, Bethesda, Maryland, 1988.

Index

A Matter of Heff, 51

Accidents, 147

Advisory Committee on Indian health, 137

Ah-Gwah-Ching Sanitarium, 73

Alaska Native health services, history, 67-70; and Bureau of Education, 68, 70; hospitals, 69, 70; Russian influence, 68; transferred to Bureau of Indian Affairs, 69

Alaska Native health survey, 122-23

Albuquerque School of Practical Nursing, 145

Alcohol, see ardent spirits

Allotment of Indian land and health, 12, 13, 30; alcohol prohibitions, 50-53; and citizenship, 50-51; and Indian Reorganization Act, 70; land loss, 159; police powers under, 50-51; trust relationship, 51

American Indian tribal nations: Alaska Natives, 25, 40n19, 66, 98, 100, 122-123; Apache, 26; Apache, Jicarilla, 37, 42n45, 150n18; Apache, Ft. Apache (White Mountain), 92, 97, 105n21; Apache, Mescalero, 31, 42n45, 150n18; Apache, San Carlos, 20, 42n45, 92; Arapaho, 6; Blackfeet, 17n12, 20, 31, 81, 92, 94; Chasta, 5; Cherokee, 3, 8, 81, 87n34; Cherokee, Eastern, 73, 81, 92; Cheyenne, 6, 114; Cheyenne, Southern, 7; Chickasaw, 3, 8; Chippewa, 16n6, 81, 87n34, 102; Chippewa, Bad River, 98, 106n24, 110; Chippewa, Fond du Lac, 41n36; Chippewa, Leech Lake, 73; Chippewa, Red Cliff, 110; Chippewa, Red Lake, 13, 14, 41n36; Chippewa, Turtle Mountain, 31, 79, 106n28; Chippewa, White Earth, 7; Choctaw, 3, 8; Comanche, 9, 26; Creek, 3, 8; Crow, 52, 92; Elko Colony, 143; Flathead, 92; Ft. Belknap, 79; Ft. Berthold, 110, 130; Hoopa, 7, 23, 39n13, 111; Hopi, 11, 35, 42n45, 100, 115, 122, 161-162; Iroquois, 29; Kaw, 7; Kickapoo, 16n6, 51; Kiowa, 9, 26; Laguna Pueblo, 92; Mandan, 4, 5; Maricopa, 1; Menominee, 10, 11, 23, 39n13; Miami, 16n6; Mission 42n45; Mojave, 39n13; Navajo, 42n45, 47, 56, 63n21, 65, 77, 92, 93, 97, 100, 101, 103, 107n37, 111, 114, 115, 116, 117, 122, 133; Nez Perce, 6; Nisqually, 5; Omaha, 1, 4, 121; Oneida, 21; Osage, 10, 16n6; Otoe, 4, 135; Ottawa, 16n6; Paiute, 13; Paiute, Lake Pyramid, 29;

183

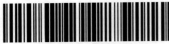

Made in the USA
San Bernardino, CA
07 January 2019